D0353975

REV UP YOUR ADULT STEM CELL POWER - YOU NEED IT NOW!

Ann M. Harrison and
Victor Neugebauer, M.D. RET.

Published by Independent Publisher, Conway Associates, Inc.

**REV UP YOUR ADULT STEM CELL POWER –
YOU NEED IT NOW!**

responsibility for author or third party websites or their content.

Independent Publisher
For information contact:
Ann M. Harrison, Conway Associates, Inc.
PO Box 17092; Clearwater, FL 33762
Phone: 727-531-7116
Or send an e-mail inquiry to:
ilovemystemcells@gmail.com

ISBN: 0615814034
First printed: May 2013

REV UP YOUR ADULT STEM CELL POWER –
YOU NEED IT NOW!

Your Co-Authors:

Ann M. Harrison has a Bachelor's and Master's Degree in Human Resources with 20+ years Pharmaceutical/ Nutritional industry experience. While working in Human Resources, at the Director level, she was responsible for providing employee services to 700+ employees, including Employee Wellness Programs. For over fifteen years Ann has been researching the subjects of complementary and alternative wellness. She has spoken to audiences of up to 300 people (professionals, medical doctors, and laymen) in various locations throughout the United States, relaying information about enhancing cellular health using natural nutrients. Ann previously had 40% gray hair – in this book she shares that she no longer has gray hair because after learning how to "tap into" the "New Fountain of Youth," her hair naturally returned to its original color.

Victor Neugebauer, M.D. RET., is a graduate of Oklahoma School of Medicine. He had a general practice and was one of the first full-time emergency room physicians in the United States. "Dr. Vic," as affectionately named by his patients, spent much of his time working in hospital emergency rooms in Florida, Georgia, Oklahoma, Vietnam, and Saudi Arabia. After 25 years, he began transitioning into retirement, and he finished out his medical career as a Ship Doctor on various cruise ships. As a result of experiencing some serious health challenges, he left the practice of medicine which opened the door to dietary supplementation, lifestyle changes and other alternative options - in this book, he shares how many of his health situations have since improved after discovering the "New Fountain of Youth."

4

With their own personal anti-aging stories and mutual appreciation for the anti-aging potential of Adult Stem Cells, Ann Harrison and Victor Neugebauer, M.D. RET. joined forces to conduct intensive research to learn more about the latest scientific developments occurring in Adult Stem Cell research and why celebrities including Dr. Oz, Suzanne Somers, Governor Perry of Texas, and Pope Benedict XVI are sharing information with others about the amazing role of Adult Stem Cells. With Dr. Vic and Ann interpreting scientific research coming out of a variety of sources, they provide the reader a short, easy-to-understand book, revealing how we can now take advantage of the scientific advances that have recently been brought to light that we all have a built-in natural renewal system – **the real "New Fountain of Youth".**

REV UP YOUR ADULT STEM CELL POWER –
YOU NEED IT NOW!

TABLE OF CONTENTS

REV UP YOUR ADULT STEM CELL POWER – YOU NEED IT NOW!

Acknowledgements

We want to extend our special thanks to everyone who took time out of their busy schedule to edit all or part of our book, including Bob Gallo and Elizabeth (Bethie) Swanson, Al Conway (as Star Editors); Marge Berger, Grace Boehm, Ruby Coleman, Mildred Cooper, Sara Finan, Yvonne Ford, Tom Gallo, Bennie Ingram, Joanne Koenig, Ron and Cara Imondi, Richard and Brenda Luddington, Marietta McManus, Tom Marsh, Max Maya-Griffin, Mario Santangelo, Wilfred Sergeant, Diane Shank, Nancy Strader, Garth Wunsch, and many others who were helpful to us with their suggestions and comments. Without all of your feedback and encouragement, this book could never have been possible.

FOREWORD

Throughout recorded history, there have been seekers of the legendary "Fountain of Youth," with many of those seekers placing their life at great risk as they traveled to distant lands. Turns out, all that traveling was in vain, as scientists uncovered the amazing truth that the anti-aging "Fountain of Youth" can be found within.

Not until the year 2000, did a scientific discovery occur of such significance that all of us can be on course to have our lives dramatically changed for the better. Some people are calling that discovery our personal "built-in Fountain of Youth," because of its anti-aging potential. This book is dedicated to those scientists whose efforts contributed to this life-changing discovery, and all the other scientists and medical doctors who are diligently working to "take it one-step-further" for the benefit of mankind.

Sadly, with the exception of a number of celebrities, wealthy individuals and very open-minded "early-adapters," the incredible anti-aging discovery, revealing we have a personal "built-in Fountain of Youth," is not having much impact on most of us living in today's society. Unfortunately, most of us are far too busy to even take the time to hear, read, learn about it, or even understand its potential life-changing ramifications. We're all living in a technology driven age, and our minds have become too cluttered with "information overload." It is impossible to comprehend all the information coming at us each day from so many sources like our cell phones, telephones, texts, "Tweets," iphones, iPads, iPods, Kindles, Nooks, 200+ television channels, radio, DVDs, CDs, billboards, advertisements, books, newspapers, magazines, the Internet, Facebook, electronic games, and the many solicited and non-solicited e-mails we receive every day. We are only human, right?

For those of us who can free our minds from this "information overload," there is GOOD NEWS and there ARE ANSWERS . . . steps we can take . . . some easy and relatively inexpensive. . . to get on the right side of the new-found anti-aging equation.

The information contained in this book was compiled as a result of conducting hundreds of hours of intensive Internet research including the review of many press releases, scientific studies, online videos, news articles, results of ongoing or concluded clinical trials, in addition to information uncovered by reading a number of books written by several scientists and medical doctors. You'll find this book a short, easy, "eye-opening" read. So, happy reading baby boomers - - and anyone else with an interest in looking and feeling younger. **It's our hope that you will enjoy learning how you can now take steps to anti-age yourself as revealed in the following pages.**

INTRODUCTION

This is a book about anti-aging. What is aging, anyway? *Merriam-Webster's Dictionary* defines aging as a "gradual change in an organism that leads to increased risk of weakness, disease, and death; and the overall effects of aging include reduced immunity, loss of muscle strength, decline in memory and other aspects of cognition, loss of color in the hair and elasticity in the skin." (Merriam-Webster Dictionary, Definition of Aging) Not a pretty picture.

There are now billions of adults inhabiting this planet. All of these people, spread across the world, have a multitude of beliefs and interests; some so radically different from others that from time to time wars erupt. Though, as diverse as the thoughts, beliefs and interests of these billions of people are, they likely have one universal thing in common. If given the chance, <u>ALL</u> of them would have a strong desire to slow down or reverse the aging process. Right? Wouldn't you?

The knowledge about anti-aging reported to you in this book was not known before the year 2000. As of this writing, many U.S. medical doctors, with their busy schedules, and having graduated before the year 2000, are probably unaware of the revolutionary information you will read about in this book, including information about the recently discovered "21st Century Fountain of Youth."

Unlike your parents, grandparents, and the generations that came before them, as a person living in the 21st Century and thanks to a recent scientific discovery of another "anatomical system," it is now known you have the natural ability to not only greatly improve your organ function but also to regenerate and rejuvenate your entire body, both inside and out, with your own Adult Stem Cells. (Note: <u>This book has absolutely</u> <u>**nothing** to do with the controversial Embryonic Stem</u> <u>Cells we've heard about in the news over the last</u> <u>several years. Instead, this book is about Adult Stem</u> <u>Cells and their anti-aging potential.</u>)

If you sincerely desire to look and feel younger, you absolutely need to read this book. Because if you do, and apply certain steps to enhance the abilities of this newfound rejuvenation system, you can experience, with wonderment, what it feels like to slow down or reverse the physiological aging process. With this information, you'll have the potential to reverse conditions from which you may have been suffering for years with the high probability of enjoying more mental clarity and increased energy while having a more youthful appearance. Further, not only will you be able to potentially anti-age yourself, but you will also learn how you can take steps to anti-age your pets. As such, **this relatively short book may well be** <u>**one of the most important books you will ever read**</u> **during your entire lifetime.** There is little doubt that the Spanish explorer, Ponce De Leon, who sought long and hard for the "Fountain of Youth," would have paid several bags of gold for the information contained within this book.

If you are questioning how any or all of this could be possible, before reading any further, your co-authors encourage you to take the time to go to the Internet <u>NOW</u> and watch the "Youtube" videos referenced below. Go to www.youtube.com and click on the hyperlinks below if you are reading the book electronically. Otherwise, if you are unable to activate these links, access an Internet browser, locate the keywords set off in quotation marks and underlined below, and type them on to the "Youtube" search bar:

1. "Skin Gun" at http://www.youtube.com/watch?v=7Y5H9Sasq5U (XSilverX, 2011)
2. "Oprah Finger Regrown Video" at http://www.youtube.com/watch?v=u3nl__psfBA (NewImageChannel, 2011)

Also, be sure to check out the following CBS newscast:

3. CBS "Seen at 11: Could the Next Generation Live to be 150? Experts Huge Breakthroughs in Science and Technology Could Make it a Reality."

   (Transcript and video of newscast). (CBS New York, 2012, para.1) http://newyork.cbslocal.com/2012/02/14/could-the-next-generation-live-to-be-150/

In terms of anti-aging, the above referenced videos are real "eye openers" providing a glimpse into how our lives are on course to radically change. Though, if you are unable to watch these videos now, do so later, and here's what you'll see when you do:

The first video shows a burn victim having his Stem Cells spray painted on his 2nd degree burns and, four days afterward his skin looked like it had been totally repaired. The second video shows Dr. Oz taking a tour of a "body parts factory," <u>where he saw scientists had taken someone's Adult Stem Cells to grow an entire gall bladder in only a few weeks</u>. The third shows a news report in the health section of a mainstream media outlet, which makes the case for humans being able to live until 150 years of age.

WOW!! As you can see, by viewing the above referenced videos, anti-aging is now possible for people living in the 21st Century!

Note: <u>There was **never a ban placed on Adult Stem Cell research** in the United States. President Bush placed a ban on Embryonic Stem Cell research, not Adult Stem Cell research. When President Obama lifted the ban, he lifted the ban on Embryonic Stem Cell research.</u>

In this book, we are <u>not</u> going to talk about the Embryonic Stem Cells a fetus has. Instead, we are going to talk about Adult Stem Cells that are released from our bone marrow every day since the day of our birth. You may want to take a look at <u>the first six minutes</u> of a U.S. based medical doctor's informational "Youtube" video by Dr. Christopher Centeno of Regenerative Sciences entitled: *What's the Difference between Embryonic and Adult Stem Cells?* (Centenohome, 2007). This video can provide you a better understanding of how your Adult Stem Cells can benefit you every day.

It is a fact that the discovery of the amazing power of Adult Stem Cells is going to change the world as we know it. In an article that appeared in the April 8, 2012, edition of *The Hindu Business Line*, "The global Stem Cell therapy market was pegged at $21 billion in 2010. It is projected to grow to $60 billion by 2015, according to a study by YES Bank and the Federation of Asian Biotech Associations (FABA)." (soma@thehindu. co.in, 2012, para. 3) We should all be holding our Adult Stem Cells in the highest regard; it is our Adult Stem Cells that are keeping us alive, and our Adult Stem Cells can anti-age us as well. (Though, as you will learn later in this book, the amount of our circulating Adult Stem Cells declines with age.)

Because it is becoming more widely known that Adult Stem Cells play a crucial role in optimal health, celebrities have been making appearances to educate the public about the role of Adult Stem Cells. Over the last few years, with more people becoming aware of Adult Stem Cells and their restorative abilities, tens of thousands of people worldwide have taken Stem Cell Therapy.

Before proceeding to Chapter 1 of our book, we want to remind you of the expression, "You can lead a horse to water, but you can't make it drink (think)." **If you are really serious about discovering how to anti-age yourself, you must make a concentrated effort to "think outside the box" as you learn about the**

scientifically proven role of Adult Stem Cells. Why? Because studies show that once a new scientific discovery is made, it normally takes at least 17 years (some say it often takes as long as 25-40 years) before the general population accepts a radically new concept. To bring this to light, "Penicillin was discovered by Sir Alexander Fleming in 1928. However, not until 17 years later, in 1945, was Penicillin commercially available." ("Who discovered Penicillin?," 2012) Think of all the hundreds of thousands of people who needlessly died of bacterial infections, including the many soldiers who died during World War II, during that 17 year period. It is very sad, isn't it?

Let us provide another example about people being slow or resistant to changing their mindset: In an article written by Paul Altrocchi, M.D., entitled "Ideational Change: Why is it so difficult to Change?" Dr. Altrocchi relayed: "For four decades I have watched MDs switch immediately to new antibiotics and new gadgetry like MRI scanning, yet the same MDs would maintain outmoded concepts for their entire career, putting the very lives of their patients in jeopardy. As a physician, I have witnessed both crippling and death on a number of occasions by outworn MD ideas and steadfast refusal to change." (Altrocchi, M.D.)

Unfortunately, studies have shown that many of us are very close-minded and we are extremely resistant to

15

change, even if it is for our own good. Your co-authors sincerely hope you are not one of the masses who resist change and that you will be the exception to the rule. Because if you can open your mind and begin to understand the role of your Adult Stem Cells – the "New Fountain of Youth" - and integrate this revolutionary, life-changing concept into your mindset, then you can clearly understand <u>why</u> and <u>how</u> you indeed have the potential to begin <u>anti-aging</u> yourself starting TODAY.

CHAPTER 1 – (THE FOUNTAIN OF YOUTH/MY PERSONAL STORY)

If you are like us and over age 55, well, we're glad we made it this far. Through the grace of God and good luck, we have avoided disasters like being hit by a bus, losing our life to a terrible disease, or succumbing to a massive heart attack. Yes, the good news is that we are still "alive and kicking."

The bad news is, if you are like many of us baby boomers or seniors, your body just "ain't what it used to be." As a result, many of us don't like what we see in the mirror, do we? And, like many in our age group, we just don't like what our bodies are feeling – things we've never felt before in our younger days. You know what I mean – in places like knees, fingers, hips, and in other places we never knew we could feel such discomfort. Even our grandparents couldn't have prepared us for what we feel in these aging bodies. Despite all this discomfort, most of us should consider ourselves lucky if we compare ourselves to many others we see hobbling down the street – for me, it's just plain frightening. When I take a trip to the store, and stop to take time to notice so many others in our age bracket walking by – I am amazed to see so many people having difficulty walking – so many using canes, walkers and wheelchairs, or so many walking unassisted with a dramatically apparent limp. Conventional treatments have not brought satisfactory results to the people we see who are obviously suffering from mobility problems. But, all those mobility problems ultimately inspired us to write this book.

You may be interested to know that over the last year, I (Ann) have been in the process of "turning back the hands of time" and anti-aging myself. Instead of looking older with each passing month, friends have been saying I have been looking younger. I have been anti-aging myself on the inside, as evidenced by me having more energy and increased mental clarity. I have also been anti-aging myself on the outside - not only does my skin have a younger appearance, but my hair does also. For example, over a year and a half ago at least 40% of my hair was gray. Today, I have no signs of gray hair remaining; because, over the last recent months, my hair returned to its original color. I did not dye or tint my hair to return it to its natural color, it all changed back to its original color on its own (as a result of taking two nutritional capsules per day, which we will later explain – although, please realize the nutritional capsules mentioned are only a very small part of the subject matter of this book – the primary subject of this book is the anti-aging potential of Adult Stem Cells).

As my hair was being restored to its original color, some of my friends decided to follow my lead and have similarly been looking younger. Nicely enough, a number of my friends have also been noticing significant improvements from conditions that they had been suffering from for years. For example, many of my friends have been witnessing improvements with their joints, mobility, skin, mental clarity, and various other situations (as revealed by conventional medical tests). During recent months, a number of my friends' faces are now looking less wrinkled, and I have noticed their eyes are brighter, their complexions are rosier, and some even have more hair on their head than before. Like my friend Mildred, some have regained their confidence in their agility, leading them to decide to dust off their high-heels and dance again. Wow! Pretty incredible, isn't it? What I enjoy the most about these amazing changes in my friends is watching the gleam in their eyes and the smiles on their faces when they recount the changes they have personally experienced with others.

As a result of experiencing such positive changes, some of these people have told me they now feel "like they have their life back."   Other people have told me they feel like they have a new-found purpose in life. In addition, one of my friends summarized her thoughts in an e-mail to me after listing all the wonderful changes she has recently been experiencing, concluding her e-mail with the following words: "In short, life is pretty grand now."

HOW I LEARNED ABOUT THE "21st CENTURY FOUNTAIN OF YOUTH"

For me (Ann), it all started to become clear in May of 2011. After having taken 2 very unique nutritional capsules every day for 10 weeks, I went to visit a friend. During our get-together, my friend, who is very good at noticing people's looks and subtle changes in appearance, brought to my attention that I no longer had gray hair, and my original hair color had come back. My hair color was always mousey blonde but when I go out in the sun for long periods of time, my mousey blonde hair turns to light blonde in certain areas – and, you know sometimes it is difficult to tell the difference between light blonde from gray when the two hair colors are interspersed. Oddly enough, about four months prior to my friend pointing out my hair color change, I was very much aware that at least 40% of my hair was gray. And, being so disheartened about all the gray I was noticing in my hair, one day I looked in the mirror and said aloud to myself, "Face it

Ann, you are going to have totally gray hair, just like your mother." I said that to myself as a form of a "self talk" to help me adjust to what I thought, at the time, was inevitable – that someday I would have all gray hair. So, after my friend pointed out I had no more gray hair, I immediately returned home to ask my husband to look at my hair. He, then, carefully looked at my hair, using his fingers to methodically separate the strands on the top of my head as he stared intently at the crown of my head, and he said "Your friend is right, you no longer have gray hair."

Now, I ask you, how many people have you known during your entire lifetime that had their hair color naturally restored to its original color, without the use of hair dyes or tints? Zero, right? So, have we piqued your interest in learning more? We hope so.

PASSIONS AND INTERESTS

You may be wondering, who are the co-authors of this book called *Rev Up Your Adult Stem Cell Power – You Need It Now?* Each of us is pretty much a person like you. Similar to most people, we enjoy our passions and hobbies. Some people may have a passion for cooking, golfing, going on "Facebook," or doing something else that "makes their heart sing." And, if you have been fortunate to have enough time to live your passion, you might be aware that those who have the time to do so, can eventually become somewhat of an expert about their passionate subject, can't they?

With my (Ann's) background being Human Resources, Employee Training, Communications and Employee Benefits (including Employee Wellness), I ultimately developed a passion for researching complementary and alternative wellness subjects, including anti-aging and nutritional supplementation. Then, as a result of conducting this type of research, if I come across information I believe could prove helpful to others, I love passing that information along. For the last 15+ years, I have been focusing on this passion, and over the last couple years, I have been focusing on some things that are really "cutting-edge." And, one of those "cutting-edge 21st Century subjects" led me to learn about the very unique nutritional capsules I have been taking that ultimately resulted in my gray hair returning to its original blonde color.

HOW MY OWN STORY BEGAN
Let me tell you how my personal story began and how I originally found out about these amazing nutritional capsules 10 weeks before I had learned my original hair color had been naturally restored.

It all started because I was attempting to help some friends by conducting intensive Internet research. My friends had expressed an interest in wanting an OTC (over-the-counter) cold light level laser device (an F.D.A. registered hand held device, which emits a warm, gentle light and photons to enhance cellular function) I had previously purchased for myself for home use. They were unwilling to spend as much money as I had invested to purchase the laser, so I thought I would see what else was on the market that was less expensive. I searched the Internet off-and-on for weeks, and one day I spotted another OTC cold light level laser listed on a website. So, I phoned the person advertising the laser, and she said, "I have been selling this particular laser for about six years now. I previously used the laser on myself all the time, but I hardly use it now, because I can pretty much get the same results by taking some nutritional capsules." Of course, I replied, "Tell me more." That is how I learned about the wonderful nutritional capsules that ultimately led to the restoration of my original hair color within 10 weeks.

During the conversation I had with the lady selling the laser, she suggested I speak to her 73 year old mother, a nutritionist, living in Florida. As a result of speaking with her mother, I arranged to meet her, along with one of her friends, a lady who was 71 years old, who had been taking the nutritional capsules. When I met these two older women for the first time, I was amazed at how much more energy they seemed to have than I did at the time and also, how much more active both of these women were (back then) compared to me. Whereas many people their age would have been content to be 100% retired, both of these women were still going strong. For example, the younger of the two ladies is still managing more than a dozen rental properties, which she and her husband own – and, when one of their tenants vacate, she will repaint the walls and do all that's necessary to ready the rental property for the next tenant. The lady who was 73 years old still plays tennis and recently told me she is running each day to get in shape to run in an upcoming marathon (senior category). She also works out in the gym, and can now bench press as much as her body weight. When I met these two ladies for the first time, and saw all the energy they were exuding while being at least 13-15 years older than me, I wondered, how could they have so much more energy than myself, when they were so much older than me? That is when I decided to try the nutritional capsules they were taking. With what I know now, I believe that was one of the best decisions I have ever made in my life.

BACK IN THE GAME

More about these unique nutritional capsules: (The nutritional capsules I am referring to influence my bone marrow to release more Adult Stem Cells into blood circulation. Note: The nutritional capsules did not cause my hair to return to its original color, but an increased number of Adult Stem Cells in my blood circulation did. Later in this book, you will learn why having an increased number of Adult Stem Cells in blood circulation can be very beneficial.) I know quite a number of people who have been taking the same kind of nutritional capsules I am taking. By talking with these people, I have learned one thing for certain: each one of us taking the capsules experiences different results. This is because every person's body is different. When I started taking these nutritional capsules, I felt by the third day a noticeable change in three areas:

1. Increased mental clarity;

2. Increased energy level; and,

3. Feeling far less stressed

As a result, I felt "I had my life back" and that I was "back in the game." Why? Primarily because, by Day 3, I felt that the "brain fog," I had been experiencing for several years, had lifted. Now, some women might know what I am talking about when I mention "brain fog." It's what I have come to understand as something many of us baby boomer women feel as a result of changes in our hormones (i.e. menopause). When these changes in hormones occur, for some reason women sometimes do not seem to be able to process information like they used to; it is almost like having the feeling of not being able to grasp things quickly, or having things occur that "go over our head." It's difficult to describe, but many women who have gone through menopause might be able to relate to my experience of "brain fog." When my "brain fog" feeling disappeared, my self-confidence improved. With increased mental clarity, I regained the ability to process information more quickly, similar to what I had been able to do years before.

Yes, as a result of the positive changes I experienced after starting my daily capsule regime, I feel so blessed that I learned about these Adult Stem Cell enhancer nutritional capsules last year, rather than finding out about their existence sometime in the far distant future. (NOTE: For those who may have an interest in knowing the brand name of the Adult Stem Cell enhancer nutritional capsules that gave me such positive results, this will be covered later in this book.)

ENCOURAGING A FRIEND

After starting to take the Adult Stem Cell enhancer nutritional capsules for a few weeks, I happened to telephone a friend of mine, named Ruby, who is a professional entertainer/singer, and I learned from her that she basically hadn't had the gumption to "get up and go" for three days because she was in a "funk." I knew why she was in a "funk:" after being a full-time professional entertainer for over 30 years, she had basically run out of the intense physical energy that is required to maintain the non-stop schedule often associated with being a professional entertainer. And, because of that energy requirement, most anytime I spoke with her, she was constantly expressing her desire to retire from show business. So, learning that she was feeling so blue, I said everything I could think of to cheer her up and convince her to get out of her house and rejoin civilization. As a form of enticement, I asked her to meet my husband and me at a local restaurant, and I suggested that she also bring her husband along. Fortunately, something I said "did the trick," and she agreed to meet us for lunch. Soon, thereafter, when my husband and I walked into the restaurant, we saw my entertainer friend and her husband sitting in a booth. When we came over to their table, I noticed her husband had a surprised look on his face as he watched us walking toward them. Then, he leaned over toward his wife, Ruby, and whispered something into her ear. (Prior to that day, we had been socializing with this couple on a fairly regular basis over the last 18 months, so they had come to know us fairly well, including our demeanors, appearance and respective energy levels.) As soon as we sat down, her husband asked me, "What are you doing? You look so different!" Before I could respond, he went on to say that as professional entertainers with their demanding schedule, it took a considerable amount of energy. He further added the two of them had often found it necessary to regularly take some "pick-me-uppers," such as strong aspirin and caffeinated energy drinks, etc., to keep up with their demanding schedule. He admitted that some of those things, if taken on a long term basis, had known adverse side effects. He then said, "There is a remarkable improvement in your overall appearance and energy level. When I saw you walking over to our table, I told Ruby that whatever Ann is doing, we are going to do it too." (And, this from a man who often encourages his wife not to spend money on unnecessary things for reasons of being budget conscious.) Of course, I proceeded to tell him about what I had done to experience such positive changes.

So that, my baby boomer friends, is how it all got started. After noticing such positive effects – feeling more energized, with improved mental clarity, feeling far less stressed - simply by adding two very unique nutritional capsules to my daily regime, you can bet I made the decision to keep taking those very special capsules. And, as Paul Harvey would say, "Now, for the rest of the story...."

CHAPTER 2 - (OUR NATURAL RENEWAL SYSTEM)

THE SECRET REVEALED–OUR NATURAL RENEWAL SYSTEM

What is the secret behind the nutritional capsules that dramatically improved my energy level, mental clarity, and led to my original hair color being restored? Why had my friend's budget-conscious husband noticed such a marked change in my appearance to the point that he was willing to spend money on the same thing I was doing? The secret behind these nutritional capsules is they influenced my "Natural Renewal System" to bounce back and work more effectively.

OUR NATURAL RENEWAL SYSTEM: OUR STEM CELL SYSTEM

"Just as we have numerous anatomical systems in our body like a Digestive System, and a Cardiovascular System, it is now known that we have a "Natural Renewal System" of our body – our Bone Marrow Adult Stem Cell System, which constitutes the repair system of the body, and, for our survival, supports all our other anatomical systems." (Paraphrased) (Drapeau, MSc, 2010, p. 55-56) "Adult Bone Marrow Stem Cells can repair any injury (in our body) in the liver, kidneys, brain, heart, lungs, bone, etc., whenever they (our organs or tissues) are damaged by disease or injury. This is new science, and this information wasn't even known prior to the year 2000." (Paraphrased) (Nocera, M.D., 2011, p. 20, 23-24) As discovered in the beginning of the 21st Century, our "Natural Renewal System" is an incredible anti-aging system, and can serve as your very own internal "Fountain of Youth."

A MEDICAL DOCTOR'S OPINION ABOUT STEM CELLS
To bring to light how magnificent our Stem Cells are, let's take a look at what a medical doctor relayed to us in *the Atlantic* magazine on January 19, 2012: Leo Furcht, M.D., Chairman of the Department of Laboratory Medicine and Pathology at the University of Minnesota Medical School, writing in conjunction with William Hoffman, editor and writer for 25 years, relayed, "Stem Cells are proving to be the silver bullet, and the Holy Grail...They could alleviate ALL manner of suffering, whether it's caused by disease, injury or genetic fate...they have the power to regenerate tissue that is healthy and repair tissue that is diseased or damaged." Thank you very much, Dr. Leo Furcht, (M.D.) and William Hoffman for publishing your article in *the Atlantic* magazine so we baby boomers and the general public can get a better understanding of the amazing power of our Stem Cells. It is good to know that a very well-respected U.S. medical doctor has gone on record as saying that **Stem Cells could alleviate "ALL manner of suffering,"** from the article entitled, "The Holy Grail of Medicine: On the Mystery and Power of Stem Cells." (Furtch/Hoffman, 2012, para. 7)

ANOTHER MEDICAL DOCTOR'S OPINION ABOUT ADULT STEM CELLS:
As Christopher J. Centeno, M.D., relayed in a "Youtube" video posted on August 3, 2007, entitled, *What is the Difference between Embryonic Stem Cells*

and Adult Stem Cells? - "Adult Stem Cells are the body's repair cells, and this is really rewriting medicine for the 21st Century. As a result, textbooks will have to be re-written." (Centenohome, 2007)

Think about Dr. Christopher Centeno's prediction. If textbooks will need to be rewritten because of the newly discovered role of Adult Stem Cells, what better time to learn more about your Adult Stem Cells than now?

DID YOU KNOW YOU HAVE GREAT NUMBERS OF ADULT STEM CELLS?

Since birth, your bone marrow has been sending out great numbers of Adult Stem Cells into your blood circulation every day. Scientists and medical doctors have known about Adult Stem Cells for at least 40 years. You have heard of bone marrow transplants, haven't you? For over 40 years, scientists and medical doctors were aware Adult Stem Cells come out of our bone marrow every day; and, Adult Stem Cells could change to become red blood cells, platelets and white blood cells. Isn't it incredible that Adult Stem Cells have the ability to change to become different types of cells in our body? Their ability to change into different types of cells is known as "pluripotency." Yes, it was known for several decades that our Adult Stem Cells could change to become red blood cells, white blood cells, and platelets, but that was just about all that was known about the role of Adult Stem Cells for 40 years. (Gupta, Johns Hopkins Medicine)

LIFE-CHANGING DISCOVERY MADE IN THE YEAR 2000!!!!
In the beginning of the 21st Century, a phenomenal scientific discovery was made – a discovery that the Adult Stem Cells, which come out of our bone marrow in great numbers every day, can change to become other types of specialized cells in our body. Our body has about 220 different specialized cells. (Wikipedia fact-index, 220 types of cells)

According to *Medical News Today*, "Adult Stem Cells exist throughout the body after embryonic development and are found inside your bone marrow and different types of tissue. Adult Stem Cells can divide or self-renew indefinitely, enabling them to generate a range of cell types from the originating organ or even regenerate the entire original organ. (Medical News Today, {n.d.})

You name it, and your Adult Stem Cells can change into it. Similar to how a master key can open any lock, Adult Stem Cells can become any type of specialized cell. Or, to provide another analogy: Like a talented sculptor who can shape a ball of clay to take the appearance of any object, your Adult Stem Cells are able to do the same thing at the cellular level because your Adult Stem Cells have the ability to virtually change into any type of cell in your body.

Adult Stem Cells are not only "Master Cells," with the ability to change into any type of specialized cell in your body, incredibly, they are also "Smart Cells." They are considered "Smart Cells" because, as scientists and medical doctors theorize, they know what to repair in order of importance, and they will fix your life threatening situations before they fix the non-life threatening situations.

When Adult Stem Cells change to become different types of specialized cells, they multiply many times over and change to become the same type of specialized cells your body needs for repair purposes. For example, if you were to sustain a heart attack, in simplistic terms, the Adult Stem Cell repair process would occur something like:

1. In regard to your hypothetical heart attack, in order to save your life, your heart would send out biochemical S.O.S. signals into your blood.
2. Your Adult Stem Cells in your bone marrow would receive the S.O.S. signals.
3. In response, your Adult Stem Cells in your bone marrow would begin mobilizing.
4. Having multiplied many times over, <u>including each one making a sister cell to leave behind</u>, your Adult Stem Cells would exit the bone marrow into your blood. (With each Adult Stem Cell leaving a duplicate or a "sister cell" behind, you don't have to worry that your bone marrow will run out of Adult Stem Cells just because they would be leaving your bone marrow to fix your area of distress.)
5. Then, once in your blood circulation, your Adult Stem Cells would home in on additional

biochemical S.O.S. signals being sent from the affected area and travel to your hypothetical injured heart.

6. Once entering the distressed area of your heart, your Adult Stem Cells would again multiply many times over, making more copies of themselves as Adult Stem Cells.

7. Then, once they have multiplied in your heart to great numbers, your Adult Stem Cells would change to become heart cells to repair the damaged heart cells that resulted from your hypothetical heart attack. (Paraphrased) (Drapeau, MSc, 2010, p. 111-112)

Note: If you had much more than a sufficient amount of Adult Stem Cells going to your heart, "full repair and formation of functional tissue would take place. However, if not enough Stem Cells are available for full repair, scarring would then take place in order to bring the body to homeostasis as soon as possible." (Drapeau, MSc, 2010, p. 200) Older people who sustain a heart attack would likely end up having a significant amount of scar tissue after incurring a heart attack; because, as a result of their age, they would probably not have a sufficient amount of Adult Stem Cells available to effectively repair their heart. The more Adult Stem Cells sent to fix the problem heart, the better.

Aren't your Adult Stem Cells amazing? Their role is to rejuvenate your body. Your Adult Stem Cells serve as an "all-natural built-in repair kit." This is all new science! How was the remarkable role of Adult Stem Cells discovered that was kept secret from man for centuries? The secret was uncovered in the year 2000, when scientists observed that bone marrow cells from a rat and human had changed to become neurons. "Rat and Human Bone Marrow Stomal Cells Differentiate Into Neurons." (Woodbury D, Schwarz EJ, Prockop DJ, and Black IB, 2000)

Then, in 2001, scientists induced a mouse to have a heart attack. Afterward, they stained some bone marrow Stem Cells from the mouse the color green, using a Green Fluorescent Protein, which had been taken from a jellyfish. Then they injected the mouse's green-stained bone marrow Stem Cells back into the mouse, near the location of the mouse's heart. Days later, the scientists looked at the mouse's heart and noticed that some of the mouse's heart cells were green. Since the scientists had never placed green heart cells in the mouse's heart, the scientists determined that the only way the mouse could have green heart cells was if the bone marrow Adult Stem Cells, which had been stained green, had migrated to the mouse's heart and then after traveling to the site of the heart, they changed from green bone marrow Adult Stem Cells to green heart cells. Reference: PubMed.gov Abstract, "Bone Marrow Cells Regenerate Infarcted Myocardium." (Orlic D, Kajstura J, Chimenti S, Jakoniuk I, Anderson SM, Li B ..... Anversa P., 2001)

REV UP YOUR ADULT STEM CELL POWER –
YOU NEED IT NOW!

(Note: Since the role of Adult Stem Cells is considered so significant, and the discovery was made possible because of the Green Fluorescent Protein, the Japanese scientists who had previously discovered the Green Fluorescent Protein in 1964 were justly awarded the Nobel Prize in Chemistry in 2008. If you are interested in learning more information about these Nobel Prize winners and their scientific discovery, you may want to access the Internet yourself including looking through the archives of www.nobelprize.org.)

ADULT STEM CELLS ARE IN THE NEWS
Thanks to the news media, we in the United States have recently been hearing and reading more about Adult Stem Cells:

During 2011, several celebrities were seen on the media educating people about Adult Stem Cells including Dr. Oz and Oprah. In December 2011, Suzanne Somers announced on an Internet talk show that she took Adult Stem Therapy for purposes of breast reconstruction. In the news media, we learned that one of our esteemed athletes, Peyton Manning, traveled overseas to have Adult Stem Cell Therapy for his neck. Perhaps you may have seen on the nightly news or "Youtube" some featured stories about women getting Adult Stem Cell facelifts performed by their plastic surgeons, or dogs getting Adult Stem Cell Therapy by their veterinarians for joint problems.

During a September 2011 South Carolina town hall meeting, when Governor Perry was asked about Stem Cell research, Governor Perry spoke about his own back surgery that used Stem Cells: "I am a huge Adult Stem Cell proponent," he said. "My recovery has been just fascinating. ... I hope all of you will educate yourselves as much as possible about Adult Stem Cells." (Schultheis, 2011, para. 6)

In November 2011, Pope Benedict XVI publically spoke out in favor of Adult Stem Cell research during a three day International Adult Stem Cell Conference held at the Vatican City, which was attended by 250 carefully selected people, including scientists, medical doctors and Stem Cell experts from around the world. (Romereports, 2011) You may be interested to know that in Amazon.com's bookstore, you should be able to find information about a Vatican endorsed book focusing on Adult Stem Cells entitled <u>The Healing Cell</u> with a message in the book written by Pope Benedict XVI. The Vatican even donated one million dollars to start a non-profit organization, called the "Stem for Life Foundation," to focus on Adult Stem Cell education campaigns and research in collaboration with a New York Adult Stem Cell company called NeoStem. (Taylor, 2011, para. 1)

On May 9, 2011, ABC News featured a story about a woman who took Adult Stem Cell Therapy for her joints: "Hoping to avoid surgery, Patricia Beals, 72, opted instead for experimental treatment that involved harvesting bone marrow Stem Cells from her hip, concentrating the cells in a centrifuge and injecting them back into her damaged joints. Ms. Beals relayed, **'Almost from the moment I got up from the table, I was able to throw away my cane. Now, at age 72, I'm biking and hiking like a 30-year-old'.**" (Neporent, 2011, para. 3) Now, I ask you, isn't that incredible?

REV UP YOUR ADULT STEM CELL POWER –
YOU NEED IT NOW!

If you live in California, you may have seen NBC's televised news report in August, 2011, revealing that some people are paying over $500 to have Adult Stem Cells removed from the pulp of freshly extracted teeth and placed in "cold storage" for potential future use. "The Stem Cells in teeth are called Mesenchymal cells, and they form tissues such as nerves, blood vessels, muscles, including heart muscles," said oral surgeon Jay Reznick." (Lin, 2011, para. 3)

Speaking about "cold storage," over the last several years, if you became a parent (or grandparent), you might have been encouraged by a hospital representative or medical doctor to cryo-preserve your newborn's Adult Stem Cells (from the umbilical cord or placenta) for possible future use.

Or, perhaps you read through the March 18, 2013 online edition of *Esquire magazine* and saw a photo of a cryogenic tank displayed in the article entitled, "Whatever Happened to Stem Cells?" with a caption appearing underneath the photo reading: "Cryogenic tank at Dr. Anthony Atala's lab at Wake Forest, capable of holding 100,000 samples of stem cells, a store theoretically big enough to grow organs for 90 percent of the population." (Cabot, 2013, p. 1) What? 90 percent of the population! Wow! Think about that statement and the potential ramifications. I am so glad I am living at this exciting time in history and to be able to witness the beginning of the "Stem Cell Age." – Aren't you?

It was reported in 2011 that "over 50,000 people are treated around the globe each year with Adult Stem Cells" with many of these people getting their therapies outside the United States. (Prentice, Ph.D., 2011, para. 3) Predictions are that sometime within the next 10 years, the use of Stem Cell Therapy in the United States will be as prevalent as cell phone towers are today. This could happen sooner in other countries where Stem Cell Therapies are frequently being performed. To demonstrate that this might be a real possibility, if you were to go out to the Internet and access www.clinicaltrials.gov and then type in the keywords "Adult Stem Cells," you would be able to see over 4,000 Stem Cell clinical trials, which are in progress, concluded, or scheduled to start in the near future, listed on that website; or, access www.pubmed.gov and type in the search bar "Adult Stem Cells," and you will see over 35,000 scientific papers listed. Also, in 2011, a news article appeared on the Internet mentioning that there are hundreds of Stem Cell companies worldwide. As previously mentioned and worth repeating, in the April 8, 2012 edition of *The Hindu Business Line*, "The global Stem Cell therapy market was pegged at $21 billion in 2010. It is projected to grow to $60 billion by 2015, according to a study by YES Bank." (Soma@thehindu.co.in, 2012, para.3)

THE U.S. GOVERNMENT IS BANKING ON THE POWER OF ADULT STEM CELLS

A few years ago, "the U.S. Department of Defense gave a $224.7 million contract to Osiris Therapeutics (based in Maryland) for its doses of Adult Stem Cell Therapy as a medical countermeasure to nuclear terrorism and other radiological emergencies. Upon F.D.A. approval of Osiris's product (in Phase 3 Animal trials), the U.S. government will purchase at least **20,000 doses** at

$10,000 per dose. Then they will stockpile these doses in freezers around the United States." (Young, 2012, p. 7)

Now, the U.S. government would not pay $10,000 per dose (of Adult Stem Cells) if the government were not totally convinced a dose of Adult Stem Cells could have a significant positive effect on an individual who had sustained radiation poisoning. Right?

WELCOME TO THE STEM CELL AGE!
With the amazing power of Adult Stem Cells, and their ever increasing popularity as evidenced in the news media, you may be starting to realize that **we are now living in the "Stem Cell Age!"** Until recently, there has never been a time in recorded history when we could actually "anti-age" ourselves. Not until recently, did scientists and medical doctors know that Adult Stem Cells could change to become any type of cell in your body for purposes of rejuvenation. All the many generations that came before you had to suffer from physical and psychological situations for which you may now be able to avoid or reverse simply by learning how to take advantage of your Adult Stem Cell System. How exciting for us to be living in this day and age with the potential to greatly benefit from this new anti-aging science! That is, if we have an open-mind to it all.

STEM CELLS REPLACE WORN OUT CELLS

Whether or not you are aware of it, every day numerous cells in our body break down as they wear out and are replaced with other cells. You have probably heard the saying that we have a new body (on average) every seven years. The process of cells breaking down and being repaired is undetectable by us because the process is performed by our Natural Renewal System supported by our "innate intelligence," the same "innate intelligence" that we can depend upon to grow our body, keep our heart beating, and digest our food, etc. We don't consciously think "Grow my body!" "Heart, please beat!" Or, "stomach, please break down my food!" Instead, thanks to our innate intelligence, we can trust that we grow up just fine, our heart will beat, and our stomach will digest the food we eat without giving those bodily functions any thought. With large numbers of cells in our body breaking down each day, they are constantly in need for renewal and repair. As an analogy, think about it like a stock market chart. The cells breaking down in our body would be depicted like a declining line on a stock market chart. Conversely, as our cells are being repaired, the analogy would be like an increasing line on a stock market chart. Like a stock market price reflected on a stock market chart, our bodies are either in a declining mode (more cells breaking down than are being repaired) or an improving mode (more cells being renewed and repaired than are breaking down).

Taking this stock market chart analogy further, when we are very young, let's say, up through our teenage years when our Adult Stem Cells are working hard to grow our bodies, the stock market price line would be on the incline, as during that time period in our lives we have more Adult Stem Cells in our blood stream to repair and renew our body's cells than our body requires. That's the period of time in our lives when the line on the stock chart would be climbing and climbing. Then, after our teenage years, our Adult Stem Cell levels change and our stock market price line starts to even off for a number of years, and eventually, our hypothetical stock market price line starts to decline. Why? Because, on average, as we age, we have more cells breaking down than are effectively being repaired. Why? Because when we are older, we have fewer Adult Stem Cells in circulation.

GOOD NEWS FOR BABY BOOMERS – ADULT STEM CELLS CAN IMPROVE ORGAN FUNCTION

As baby boomers, many of us are aware that our organs are not functioning at an optimal level. For example, some of us have pancreatic situations as evidenced by our sugar levels, and some of us have pulmonary situations as evidenced by breathing problems. The good news is that Adult Stem Cells, with their restorative abilities, can help organ function. Like the bricks and mortar in our house, our Adult Stem Cells that change into the specialized cells of our organs can provide stability to our organs, improving organ function. **The more Adult Stem Cells we have in circulation, the better chance we have to repair and regenerate our organs and tissues**.

SOME BAD NEWS FOR BABY BOOMERS

Now for a little bit of bad news: Our body makes significantly large numbers of Adult Stem Cells every day to keep us in tip-top shape for the first part of our lives and well into our twenties. It is estimated that sometime between the ages of 30-35, our bone marrow no longer releases the required amount of Adult Stem Cells to keep us in optimal condition. And with less of these Adult Stem Cells available to constantly repair and regenerate our body, the declining amount of circulating Adult Stem Cells is not enough to keep up with our body's need to prevent aging, and this results in a reduction in overall health. With a decline in Adult Stem Cells, we cannot rebound as quickly from situations like most children can who have far more Adult Stem Cells in their blood circulation.

In October 2008, Arnold I. Caplan, Ph.D., at Case Western Reserve University, in a PowerPoint presentation, compared the estimated number of (Mesenchymal) Adult Stem Cells to Bone Marrow cells from birth to 80 years of age as follows:

(Mesenchymal) Adult Stem Cells to Bone Marrow cells:
1 in 10,000 -newborn
1 in 100,000 - teenager
1 in 250,000 - at age 30
1 in 400,000 - at age 50
1 in 2,000,000 - at age 80
(Caplan, Ph.D., Arnold, October 2008, slide 13).

As relayed by CEO Robert R. Young in the 2012 New York Stem Cell Summit Fact Sheet: "**The number of Stem Cells in a person begins declining shortly after birth. It's the decline in the number of Stem Cells that ultimately leads to wear, deterioration and, finally, death.**" ("The New York Stem Cell Summit" is a one-day (annual) event that focuses on Stem Cell therapies that are either in commercial use or will soon be in commercial use." And according to Robert R. Young, "The meeting has become the premier meeting for discussion of the emerging commercialization of Stem Cell technologies.") (Young, 2012, p. 2)

As this drop in the number of Adult Stem Cells in our blood circulation occurs, we might not even be aware that our health is on the decline. For example, if your liver, pancreas and/or heart are not being repaired by your Adult Stem Cells as efficiently as they were being repaired when you were a teenager, you probably wouldn't really notice. If during this year, the repair processes occurring in your body are only 95% as effective as last year, do you think you would notice? Probably not. Slow declines in our health over the years will probably not be detectible by most of us. (Remember the story about the frog being placed in cold water and someone gradually and slowly turned up the heat until the water started to boil? Since the change in the water temperature occurred so gradually, the frog never noticed that his life was in danger as the water was getting progressively hotter. That's why the frog did not jump out of the water. He never noticed the temperature change getting significantly hotter, since the change was so gradual.)

As revealed above, children have more Adult Stem Cells in blood circulation. Most of us are aware that, generally speaking, children do not get heart attacks. Oftentimes, it is us adults, and not children that experience heart attacks. Why do you think that is? One reason, my baby boomer friends and others interested in anti-aging, is because children have more Adult Stem Cells in blood circulation than adults. Having enough Adult Stem Cells in blood circulation gives our body the ability to keep up with the demands of the heart and to keep our hearts (and other organs and tissues) functioning well.

SOME INFORMATION ABOUT HEART DISEASE

Several years ago, I (Ann) was privileged to hold the role of a Nutritional Speaker for a world-renown medical doctor who discovered "How to Reverse Heart Disease with Natural Nutrients." I traveled around the southeast United States, speaking in front of audiences of up to 300 attendees. As a result of studying the medical doctor's materials, I learned quite a bit of information about heart disease. As relayed in his books, I learned that from time to time people's arterial walls may develop cracks ("something like a mild form of scurvy which can be caused by a Vitamin C deficiency"). (Rath, M.D., 2001, p. 44) If, by chance, a crack in our arterial wall were to occur, our body instinctively knows that these cracks, if not immediately repaired, could create a life threatening situation. What do you think the first line of defense would be to patch up a crack in your arterial wall? Yes, your arterial wall cells and your Adult Stem Cells. If you had enough Adult Stem Cells in blood circulation, then your Adult Stem Cells could travel to the crack in your artery, arrive at the scene of the damage, duplicate themselves many times over and then change into arterial wall cells to patch up and repair that crack. That (using arterial wall cells and Adult Stem Cells to patch up the crack) would be your body's first-choice line of defense to repair the crack in your artery.

ADULT STEM CELLS, ARTHEROCLEROSIS AND HEART DISEASE

Now, if you were a child experiencing a crack in the arterial wall, chances are, as a much younger person, you would have more than enough Adult Stem Cells in blood circulation to repair the crack. But because our Adult Stem Cell count declines with age, if you are an older person or a baby boomer, there is a very good chance that you would not have enough Adult Stem Cells on hand to repair that crack. And, if you didn't have enough Adult Stem Cells, your innate intelligence would work to alert your liver to send something else to repair the damaged area to patch up that crack, and most probably, that would be cholesterol. Cholesterol is sticky stuff that is really good for patching up arterial wall cracks. And, over time, if you continued to not have enough Adult Stem Cells on hand to repair your arterial wall cracks as they developed, and your body kept patching up these cracks with cholesterol, the gradual build-up of cholesterol would eventually develop into atherosclerosis (cholesterol plaque build-up), resulting in a narrowing of the arteries. Narrowing of the arteries is the reason why many of us baby boomers end up having high blood pressure, because the heart has to work a lot harder pumping blood through cholesterol laden narrowed arteries as compared to squeaky clean arteries that don't have cholesterol build-up or plaque. (Paraphrased) (Rath, M.D., 2001, p. 44)

If you were to read Dr. Roger Nocera's book, *Cells That Heal Us From Cradle To Grave*, he would tell you there is a fairly non-invasive way to assess whether a person has atherosclerosis. That way is to simply take a person's Adult Stem Cell count. (Nocera, M.D., 2011, p. 36)

Similar to how doctors can measure our white blood cell count, many doctors now know how to measure our Adult Stem Cell blood count. All they need to do is take a sample of our blood and place it into a laboratory instrument that measures our Adult Stem Cell count. If you were to go on the Internet and do some searching, you should be able to find at least one company advertising their Adult Stem Cell counting services online.

Scientists and medical doctors know what an average Adult Stem Cell count should be for an individual, and they can use that average as a baseline. Dr. Nocera relays that "a high Adult Stem Cell blood count is proof that a patient's Adult Stem Cell system is keeping up with the demand for inner artery lining cell replacement and (as a consequence, that patient) will not have atherosclerosis (cholesterol build-up of plaque). But, if a patient's Adult Stem Cell count is lower than a certain number range, we can predict with confidence that the patient's natural Adult Stem Cell system has been defeated by the artery hardening disease process." (Nocera, M.D., 2011, p. 41)

Now, doesn't what Dr. Nocera relay in his book about atherosclerosis being correlated to a low Adult Stem Cell count bring to light how important it is for us to do whatever we can to increase our Adult Stem Cell count? You bet it does, or as they used to say on the television show, *Laugh-In*, "You bet your sweet bippy" it does.

In regards to heart disease, in November 2011, "results of a Phase II human clinical trial with 60 participants were presented to the American Heart Association, indicating Adult Stem Cell Therapy works for Heart Failure patients. The patients in the clinical trial received Adult Stem Cells delivered by catheter directly into their hearts on the theory that the Adult Stem Cells could stimulate the growth of blood vessels; the treatment appeared to be safe and reduced by 78 percent the rate of major adverse events -- heart attacks, cardiac death and need for artery clearing procedures -- after one year compared with patients who received the standard of care. Based on findings from this Phase II study, the companies said they expect to move into the pivotal human trials." (Berkrot/Krauskopf, 2011)

WE HAVE OUR "HEADS IN THE SAND" LIVING IN A

TECHNO WORLD

Unfortunately, in this technologically driven society, through no fault of their own, most everyone you know is far too busy in their own world to comprehend the major significance of their Adult Stem Cell Natural Renewal System, even when they read, hear or watch "T.V." spots about it.

How sad, because of information overload, so many millions of people are totally unaware that their own Adult Stem Cells, with their restorative abilities, have the potential to help them anti-age. Never throughout recorded history have we been expected to process so much information. It is ironic, technological advances led us to the discovery of the magnificent power of Adult Stem Cells, but technological advances are keeping our minds so preoccupied that many of us are unable to "tune into" one of the most important scientific discoveries ever – the Bone Marrow Adult Stem Cell System. (And, as previously mentioned, there are many others who may be able to comprehend this information, but they are too close-minded to want to learn more about this new science.) This is a discovery of such magnitude that if we took steps to learn about it and increase our Adult Stem Cell count, from an anti-aging perspective, many of us would have the potential to greatly improve the quality of our lives.

ADULT STEM CELL COUNT AFTER A STROKE
Roger Nocera, M.D. provides another example in his book, *Cells That Heal Us From Cradle To Grave*, which further demonstrates how important it is to take steps to increase your Adult Stem Cell count. (Recall: medical doctors can measure an Adult Stem count similar to how they can measure a white blood cell count.) He mentions that if someone had a stroke, and 30 days afterward, a doctor were to measure the stroke victim's Adult Stem Cell count, "If a high enough Adult Stem Cell blood count (CD34+ Adult Stem Cell blood count) has not been achieved by one month after any stroke, we can now use that objective information to predict that the patient will not recover from the stroke neurologically, whereas, if the Adult Stem Cell blood count (CD34+cell blood count) is higher than a certain value at one month after a stroke, then the patient's neurological recovery can be accurately predicted. This has now been proven." (Nocera, M.D., 2011, p. 38); (Nocera, M.D., 2011, video). Now, knowing that piece of information, you can be assured that I would want as many Adult Stem Cells in my blood

circulation as possible to ensure my chances for a satisfactory recovery from a stroke.

A "STROKE" CAN ADVERSELY IMPACT A FAMILY

A number of years ago, my (Ann's) own father had a terrible stroke. He obviously did not have enough Adult Stem Cells in circulation, because his recovery was minimal. He completely lost all recollection of 40 years of his life. And, from that day forward, his short term memory was such that he could only remember things that had occurred during the last few minutes. After his stroke, he was unable to tend to his own physical needs unassisted. His neurological recovery never occurred. You can only imagine what a strain that put on my family – it was so heartbreaking to see him in that condition, and my sister was responsible for tending to all his needs as best as she could for the remainder of his lifetime. Based upon what Roger Nocera, M.D. relayed in his book, if my father would have had enough Adult Stem Cells in circulation, he wouldn't have had such a permanent decline in his health, nor would he have had to suffer and live such a debilitating life during his last years. And, very likely, neither would my sister nor my family have had to suffer so much as we watched him in that pitiful condition from which he never recovered. If only he would have had an adequate supply of Adult Stem Cells when he had that stroke, he most likely would have been able to avert much needless suffering.

So, remember this: It is not only for the benefit of yourself that you should work to increase your Adult Stem Cell count – it is also for the benefit of the people in your lives who would be responsible to care for you if you were to experience a situation that could adversely affect your health. By having a robust and large supply of Adult Stem Cells in your body to continually repair and renew your organs (including your brain) and tissues as they break down, you will have a much better chance of avoiding or postponing potentially debilitating situations, which could place a heavy burden on your family and friends. For the sake of your family, do all you can do to increase your Adult Stem Cell count. I believe that it is the best insurance policy known to man – and, as brought to light earlier in this book, this form of "bio-insurance" policy (your Natural Renewal Adult Stem Cell System) wasn't even known until the year 2000. All of us are living at a great time: "The Adult Stem Cell Age!" Learn how to take advantage of this incredible new-found knowledge to slow down the effects of time.

THE POWER OF ADULT STEM CELLS – WE WANT MORE!

When I (Ann) think about the amazing power of Adult Stem Cells, I sometimes feel like climbing up to my rooftop to shout: "I want more, (Adult Stem Cells), I want more!" With the amazing ability of our Adult Stem Cells to rejuvenate our bodies, we all should be shouting from our rooftops: "We want more!" To help our friends, family and others, all of us should be spreading the word about this revolutionary life-changing discovery to everyone we know. Remember, "KNOWLEDGE IS POWER."

So now that <u>you know</u> how important it is to have as many Adult Stem Cells in circulation as possible for optimal health and anti-aging purposes, let's explore four different approaches people are taking to increase their own Adult Stem Cell count. Those approaches are:

- Stem Cell Therapy
- Adult Stem Cell Enhancer Capsules
- Regular and Intensive Exercise
- Hand Held Cold Light Level Laser

CHAPTER 3 - (STEM CELL THERAPY)

STEM CELL THERAPY:

One of the four approaches you may wish to consider is taking Stem Cell Therapy. Many people are proclaiming exceptional results after taking Stem Cell Therapy. (Stem Cell Therapies can be somewhat expensive, so keep in mind there are less expensive alternatives we will learn about later in this book.)

In recent years, as you may have occasionally seen on television, some people have been traveling outside the country to get Stem Cell Therapy. People taking Stem Cell Therapy are getting Stem Cell injections, IV's (Intravenous) or implants of Stem Cells into their body. These Stem Cells are either autologous (from self) or allogeneic (from another source). In terms of Stem Cells, autologous means "from self," in other words, your own Stem Cells taken from your own body. For example, your doctor could obtain your Adult Stem Cells from your blood, fat (through means of a mini-liposuction), or bone marrow. This would be in contrast to allogeneic, which means Stem Cells taken from another person (or animal). Some sources of allogeneic Stem Cells, for example, would be from someone else's fat, blood, bone marrow, or umbilical cord.

In recent years, tens of thousands of people have taken Stem Cell Therapy in foreign countries. Many of those therapies were likely allogeneic Stem Cell Therapies. And, many U.S. citizens traveled outside the country to get those therapies because, as of this writing, the F.D.A. has not approved most of those types of Stem Cell Therapies to be performed in the United States. (Similar to the F.D.A. giving their approval to market a prescription drug, the F.D.A. does not want to give approval to Stem Cell Therapies until such therapies have been proven to be safe and effective by means of human clinical trials.) There are a few clinics in the United States that have been granted F.D.A. approval to perform some types of Stem Cell Therapies.

Today, the F.D.A. generally allows veterinarians to perform Adult Stem Cell Therapies using "minimally manipulated" Adult Stem Cells on animals in the United States.

Also, under strict guidelines, the F.D.A. generally allows Adult Stem Cell Therapies to be performed in the United States on humans if autologous (from self) Adult Stem Cells are "minimally manipulated" before being re-injected back into the body. Most commonly, the type of Adult Stem Cell Therapies being performed in the United States meeting F.D.A. approval are for cosmetic and aesthetic reasons.

A BIT OF CLINICAL SCIENCE
Your Adult Stem Cells would most likely be considered "minimally manipulated" by the F.D.A. if they were extracted from your body, and if, within a relatively short period of time (i.e. within a few hours), they were re-injected back into your body. For example,

the step-by-step process of re-injecting your own "minimally manipulated" Adult Stem Cells might be as follows:

1. Your doctor would obtain Adult Stem Cells from either your fat (taken from your belly or hip), your blood, or your bone marrow. If taken from your fat, the doctor would perform a "mini-liposuction" to extract several ounces of fat from your body.
2. Then, the doctor (or laboratory assistant) would place your extracted fat or blood in a centrifuge* to separate the Adult Stem Cells from the extracted material.
3. Then, he would also take a few ounces of your blood, and centrifuge your blood to obtain Plasma Rich Protein (PRP) from your blood. Plasma Rich Protein (PRP) contains about 10 different growth factors that stimulate Adult Stem Cells into action.
4. Then, he would mix your Adult Stem Cells with the PRP (Plasma Rich Protein).
5. To help reactivate or increase the number of your Adult Stem Cells after they are taken from your body, your doctor might choose to shine an LED or cold light level laser over the Adult Stem Cells.
6. Then, your physician would reinsert your Adult Stem Cells back into your body by I.V. injection or an implant.

The below referenced "Youtube" video, produced by a company called Adistem, shows a hypothetical Adult Stem Cell Therapy presented in an animated format:
http://www.youtube.com/watch?v=zGP8hxr395M
(AdistemVideos, 2010)

*(A centrifuge is a laboratory instrument that can separate substances of different densities by using a high spinning action – the concept is similar to using the spin cycle on your washing machine to remove water from clothes.)

F.D.A. OVERSIGHT
As of this writing, the F.D.A. is normally <u>not</u> granting approval to U.S. based doctors to perform Adult Stem Cell Therapies using Adult Stem Cells "more than minimally manipulated," which would typically involve placing someone's Adult Stem Cells with added growth factors into a Petri dish with the intent of growing them to significant numbers over a period of days/weeks. The F.D.A. asserts that growing Adult Stem Cells in a laboratory over a period of time would be somewhat equivalent to how antibiotics are developed from cultures, like Penicillin (a F.D.A approved drug), for example.

If you choose to have Adult Stem Cell Therapy performed within the United States, we would highly recommend that you ensure that your U.S. based doctor or clinic is working within F.D.A. guidelines. (Remember, to ask if the Stem Cells will be "minimally manipulated.") If the therapy does not satisfy F.D.A. guidelines, and you went forward with the procedure, you might ultimately find yourself being taken to court by the F.D.A. Many people who have traveled to other countries to have Stem Cell Therapy have reported excellent results, including reversing all symptoms of their disease.

A CELEBRITY TAKING ADULT STEM CELL THERAPY IN THE UNITED STATES

Remember, earlier in this book, we mentioned that celebrities were educating the public about Adult Stem Cells? One such celebrity is Suzanne Somers who learned about Adult Stem Cell Therapy after experiencing breast cancer. As a result of evaluating her alternatives, she decided she wanted Adult Stem Cell Therapy in conjunction with breast reconstruction. Rather than going overseas to have Adult Stem Cell Therapy, she petitioned the F.D.A. to allow her doctor to perform the therapy in the United States. The F.D.A. ultimately granted approval. Afterward, to help others better understand the role of Adult Stem Cells, she asked someone to film her doctor performing her breast reconstructive surgery, which was later shown on an episode of *Breaking Through,* a Cafemom.com popular talk show appearing on Youtube.com. During the procedure, her breast was rebuilt with her body fat and her own Adult Stem Cells. You can watch her breast being reconstructed by her surgeon if you go to www.youtube.com and type in the words "Suzanne Somers" and "Breast Reconstruction." If you take the time to watch that graphic "Youtube," you will hear Suzanne Somers relay to the audience: "The future of Stem Cells holds medical miracles we can't even imagine." (CafeMomStudios, 2011)

VARIOUS STEM CELL THERAPIES

Below is a short representative list of diseases for which people are commonly traveling to foreign countries to obtain Stem Cell Therapy:

-Cerebral Palsy
-Congestive Heart Failure

REV UP YOUR ADULT STEM CELL POWER –
YOU NEED IT NOW!

-Multiple Sclerosis
-COPD
-Parkinson's
-Spinal Cord Injury
-ALS

To learn whether Stem Cell Therapy is being performed for certain medical conditions for which you may have an interest, simply do a keyword search on the Internet using the words: "Adult Stem Cell Therapy" and then type in the name of any disease. You may also be able to listen to testimonies of people who have traveled overseas to obtain Stem Cell Therapy by going to www.youtube.com – then type in a few keywords of your choice. But, perhaps you already know someone who has taken Stem Cell Therapy.

I happened to have met someone the other day at a Fitness Expo who told me that several years ago he had Adult Stem Cell Therapy. As part of a U.S. clinical trial, he had Adult Stem Cell Therapy for degenerative disc problems. Rather than fusing his discs together, his surgeon removed his L3, L4, and L5 discs, implanted some titanium in the spine, and then re-injected this man's own Adult Stem Cells into his body. His Adult Stem Cells then traveled to the areas of distress and went to work to actually rebuild this man's three discs. (As Dr. Oz said in the "Youtube" video we previously referenced, "If you build it, your Stem Cells will come.") The man told me that if his discs had been fused together, he would not have regained full mobility of his spine. But because his Adult Stem Cells rebuilt his L3, L4, and L5 discs, he now has full mobility and he "can even touch his toes." Aren't Adult Stem Cells amazing?

Whether Stem Cell Therapies are being performed inside or outside the United States, the therapies may be financially out of reach for many people. That is because Stem Cell Therapies would <u>not</u> typically be covered by medical insurance plans because insurance companies consider them "experimental." For this reason, without reimbursement eligibility, many people taking Stem Cell Therapies probably have fairly large bank accounts.

To bring this to light, just do a search on the Internet using the keywords "cost" or "price" and "Stem Cell Therapy." You will likely be able to locate some price lists being advertised on the Internet by clinics that are performing the Stem Cell Therapies. These clinics are in various parts of the world including, for example, Mexico and Panama. When I did a keyword search using those aforementioned words, I saw one clinic on the Internet displaying its price schedule listing Stem Cell Therapy for "Joints" at a cost of $7,500 or for "Heart" for $35,000. And, at another clinic, $59,000 for Stem Cell Therapy for "Congestive Heart Failure." (For $59,000, I learned that at one clinic, the Congestive Heart Failure patient would receive three separate injections of 100 million Stem Cells, with the injections being made one hour apart.) Now, the prices mentioned above may seem high to many, but for the people getting significant results, it is far worth the cost to them. Good health is priceless. As previously mentioned, we will provide information about more affordable alternatives to Stem Cell Therapy later in this book.

If you have a serious interest in learning more about Stem Cell Therapy, you may consider going out to the

Internet and review the materials posted on a very comprehensive Internet blog maintained by David Granovsky who, with his years of involvement in Stem Cells, has come to know some of the top Stem Cell scientists and doctors in the world. If you take time to look at his blog at www.repairstemcell.wordpress.com, you will be able to see over 1,250 Stem Cell related articles posted. On his blog, you will also be able to learn that he has authored the world's first children's book on Adult Stem Cells, entitled *SUPER STEMMYS - DORIS & THE SUPERCELLS*.

Or, if you are interested in having Stem Cell Therapy yourself, you may want to consider accessing David Granovsky's website and complete an inquiry form providing your e-mail address and specific health condition. Thereafter, within a few days, you will likely receive several e-mails sent by various clinics located around the world notifying you that their clinic can treat your specific situation while giving you their estimated charge to treat that condition.

Or, another way you could learn more about Adult Stem Cell Therapy is to consider going to the bookstore or Internet to obtain some books written by the medical doctors who have been successfully performing Stem Cell Therapies, including *Cells That Heal From Cradle To Grave,* by Roger Nocera, M.D., or, *Umbilical Cord Stem Cell Therapy,* by David Steenblock, M.S., D.O., and Anthony G. Payne, PhD. Or, you may want to start making some phone calls to people advertising Adult Stem Cell Therapies on the Internet.

Also, by speaking with people who have friends or relatives who have taken Stem Cell Therapy in foreign countries, I have learned that some people who initially had very positive results, went back to get a second treatment several years later because over time, the positive benefits they experienced declined. For example, my friend's nephew has Multiple Sclerosis. When he initially went to China for treatment for his Multiple Sclerosis, he had very favorable results. But two years later, because he had regressed, he returned to China to have the therapy performed again.

I also spoke to someone working for a company that performs Adult Stem Cell Therapy for Congestive Heart Failure at a cost of approximately $60,000 for the treatment. That person shared with me that some of their patients have had to return to have the therapy again (at another $60,000 charge) if, after their initial treatment, the patients did not change their lifestyle, including quitting smoking or getting on a regular exercise program.

I also spoke to someone else whose friend had two $100,000 Stem Cell Therapy treatments for Congestive Heart Failure (total investment $200,000), and neither treatment resulted in any noticeable benefit.

Please note, like other types of therapies, Stem Cell Therapies may have potential risks. If you are considering taking Stem Cell Therapy, ask your doctor about the possibility of any associated risks. The 50,000+ people each year who have been taking Stem Cell Therapy must have come to the conclusion that any potential risks were far outweighed by the potential benefits. For autogolous (from self) Stem

Cell Therapies, with Adult Stem Cells derived directly from a person's own blood, there is virtually no possibility for rejection. Because of this, likely one of the greatest risks a person undergoing Stem Cell Therapy would be taking is experiencing "no change."

As I previously mentioned, as of this writing, on a worldwide basis most Stem Cell Therapies are being performed in countries outside the United States. Until the F.D.A. changes that situation, unless you have a fairly large bank account and are not averse to potentially leaving your family and friends behind to travel to a foreign country, you may want to evaluate other alternatives to optimize your Adult Stem Cell count.

(If the costs mentioned above seem outside of your budget, do NOT let the relatively high prices associated with Stem Cell Therapy dishearten you. We will soon be sharing with you some information about far less costly alternatives you may want to consider to increase your Adult Stem Cell count.)

HELP OUT YOUR ADULT STEM CELLS
One theory about why some people taking Adult Stem Cell Therapy do not notice any improvements, or later regress, is they may have far too many toxins (and/or parasites) in their body. Living in our modern society, all of us have many hundreds of substances stored in our cells that did not even exist during our grandparents' time. Remember, the older we are, the more toxins we will likely have stored in our body. I have heard at least one medical doctor comment that those living in today's society should be taking steps to detoxify their body every day.

To optimize the effectiveness of your Adult Stem Cells, consider taking steps to detoxify your body from heavy metals and other toxic substances that have been gradually building up in your system over the years. As relayed in Dr. Steenblock and Anthony G. Payne's comprehensive book entitled *Umbilical Cord Stem Cell Therapy*, "Doctors in Mexico who perform Stem Cell Therapy typically insist that heavy metals such as lead, cadmium, mercury and arsenic, which are toxic to proliferating cells, should be reduced as much as possible because those metals can wreak havoc on the nerve cells in the brain and spinal cord." Steenblock and Payne go on to say that "there is a simple test known as the "DSMA challenge test" to determine the level of heavy metals in your body." (Steenblock, Payne, 2006, p. 29) and "removing impediments that might hinder the body from creating normal Stem Cells is a logical, sensible measure, which is often called "detoxification" by physicians." (Steenblock, Payne, 2006, p.119)

Also, as extracted from *Umbilical Cord Stem Cell Therapy*, "leaky gut" and "candida" "might interfere with the activity of introduced Stem Cells." (Steenblock, Payne, 2006, p.30)

Note: If you decide to take steps to detoxify yourself, do your homework, and consider consulting a professional or a physician who has experience in this area. If you do not go about it the right way, you could ultimately end up re-absorbing the toxins you are trying to eliminate and/or you could experience an adverse reaction.

Also, in terms of Adult Stem Cell Therapy, we would be remiss for not mentioning that plasma rich protein (PRP), which is naturally present in your blood (with its large number of growth factors), can play a key role with influencing your Adult Stem Cells to transform to specialized cells. Some scientific experts are puzzled as to why Adult Stem Cells differentiate, asking themselves the question: "Is it the Adult Stem Cells themselves or our Plasma Rich Protein that is the most influential in facilitating their (Adult Stem Cells) differentiation into specialized cells?"

To date, neither Dr. Vic nor I have taken Adult Stem Cell Therapy. Though, be assured, if either one of us ever discovered we had a very serious health challenge, we would be very open to consider looking into Adult Stem Cell Therapy as a possible option to address the situation.

In regards to Adult Stem Cell Therapy, and being a woman who is concerned about looking her best, I must admit I do have a fairly strong desire to eventually get an Adult Stem Cell facelift, which I have heard is relatively painless and typically provides superb, long-lasting results. Last year, I attended a cosmetic surgery seminar and met a woman who had an Adult Stem Cell facelift. Previously to that, for over 20+ years, she had been a professional landscaper, which had regularly required her to be outdoors in the hot sun. The photographs that had been taken of her face before she had an Adult Stem Cell facelift revealed she had extremely wrinkled, dark, leathery looking skin. However, when I spoke to her at the seminar, her face looked to me like she had the face of a flawless "porcelain china doll." Her face looked so beautiful with no apparent traces of ever having any type of cosmetic surgery. She was the envy of the crowd, as she looked at least 20 years younger than before. With me being able to see first-handed the phenomenal results she had, it gave me an even deeper appreciation of the incredible anti-aging powers of our (very smart) Adult Stem Cells.

For anti-aging purposes, Dr. Vic and I are currently using several less expensive approaches to increase our Adult Stem Cell count, which we will share with you in Chapters 4-6. Those three approaches include using: 1) Adult Stem Cell enhancers; 2) Regular intensive exercise; and, 3) an F.D.A. registered hand-held OTC cold light level laser.

CHAPTER 4 – (ADULT STEM CELL ENHANCERS)

CONSUME NUTRITIONAL PLANT-BASED ADULT STEM CELL ENHANCER CAPSULES
As mentioned at the start of this book, I take two nutritional plant-based capsules every day, which substantially increase my Adult Stem Cell count. The two capsules that both Dr. Vic and I take are supposed to increase the number of our circulating Adult Stem Cells by 3-4 million, within one hour of consumption. (3-4 million Adult Stem Cells is a fairly small amount compared to the numbers associated with Adult Stem Cell Therapy, where patients are typically receiving up to tens of millions of Stem Cells during their treatment.) The capsules we take are produced by a company that wants to be known as a "health sciences company" and that company has taken steps to run their nutritional products through human clinical trials to prove their effectiveness. The capsules we take

were proven in a human clinical trial to increase circulating Adult Stem Cells by 25%-30% within one hour of taking two capsules, and the results of that clinical trial were published in five medical journals, including the journal of *Cardiovascular Revascularization Medicine.* (Jensen, Hart, and Zaske, 2007) In terms of considering spending some of your money on Adult Stem Cell enhancer capsules (compared to taking Adult Stem Cell Therapy), you might be interested to know that with the nutritional capsules we are taking, we get approximately 21 million or more extra Adult Stem Cells in our blood circulation over a 7 day period (3 million/day average x 7 days = 21 million), at an approximate cost of about $13.50. (Note: For price comparison purposes, if you are a fan of the television show "60 Minutes," you may have seen a segment that revealed a representative from "60 Minutes" had ordered some Stem Cells from a Stem Cell Therapy doctor practicing in Ecuador at a cost of $5,000 for approximately 20 million Stem Cells.)

A note from Dr. Victor Neugebauer, M.D. RET.
As we age, our production and release of Adult Stem Cells into the circulation slows down and eventually nearly ceases. Younger people should benefit from higher levels of circulating Adult Stem Cells with a better immune system and more effective repair of any cellular damage and/or deterioration. For older people, it is even more important to boost the levels of circulating Adult Stem Cells. At this time there are only a few ways demonstrated to actually increase levels of circulating Adult Stem Cells. One way is by taking the Adult Stem Cell enhancer product mentioned in this book. There are other products with claims of effectiveness in increasing circulating Adult Stem Cells

levels. Some of them may actually work, but as of this date, I do not know of any other natural plant-based product that has been proven effective in scientific clinical studies on humans comparable to the Adult Stem Cell enhancer nutritional product I have been taking. I would prefer using something proven effective for myself.

CLINICAL TRIALS
Note: With me (Ann) previously being employed at a pharmaceutical/nutritional manufacturer for over 20 years, when I decide to add a nutritional product to my regime, I have a high preference for products that have been proven effective in human clinical trials. In contrast to the nutritional industry, pharmaceutical companies must successfully demonstrate to the F.D.A. that their pharmaceutical products are both:

a. Safe, and
b. Effective.

Pharmaceutical companies can prove effectiveness by successfully running their drug product through human clinical trials. (It may cost a pharmaceutical company well in excess of 50 million dollars, and as much as ten years' time, to develop a drug and eventually run that drug through Phase I-III human clinical trials.) Effectiveness is proven by "statistical significance" as a result of analyzing the results of the drug on humans during clinical trials.

In contrast to pharmaceutical companies, because nutritional products are considered "food," as of this writing the F.D.A. is not requiring nutritional companies to run their products through clinical trials to prove that nutritional products (produced from natural plants) are effective. With it being very costly to conduct a human clinical trial, very few nutritional companies ever run their nutritional products through clinical trials. Likely, less than 5% of all nutritional products on the market have been proven effective in a human clinical trial.

Any company can market a nutritional product with implications that it is effective; however, if the nutritional product was never tested and demonstrated to be effective in a human clinical trial, we are simply "running on blind faith" that the nutritional product will live up to its marketing claims. So remember, just because a nutritional product is deemed as safe, this does not necessarily mean it is effective.

When assessing the significance of the clinical trial, you will want to know if the clinical trial was either an in-vitro or an in-vivo clinical trial. In-vivo means "inside the body," such as in a human clinical trial. In-vitro means "outside the body" (like in a Petri dish or test tube). Make sure the product you are considering was run through a human clinical trial (in-vivo) and not just a clinical trial that occurred in some Petri dish (in-vitro) in a laboratory. (I have read that Stem Cells behave a lot differently in a Petri dish than they do in a human body.) If you are unable to determine if a product has been run through a human clinical trial, do not hesitate to telephone the company producing the product to ask if their company's product was proven effective by means of a human clinical trial. You should be able to find the company's phone number on the product label or by searching the Internet.

Also, because of an experience I had while working for a pharmaceutical/nutritional manufacturer, I learned the importance of placing a heavy value on clinically testing a product to prove effectiveness. Let me share that experience with you now. The company where I worked is a manufacturer of "gelcaps" (soft elastic gelatin capsules). In an effort to enhance "Employee Wellness," the company distributed a free bottle of multi-vitamins to its employees three times per year. As our company grew in size, one year the company hired a nutritionist to join the employee roster. Believing a nutritionist should know how to develop a formula for a multi-vitamin capsule better than a research chemist would, the management of the company requested the nutritionist to reformulate the product and revise the list of ingredients for the employee multi-vitamin product. The company's management made the assumption that the nutritionist would have the knowledge to improve the product formulation for the employees' multi-vitamin. The nutritionist revised the list of ingredients, removing all the minerals from the existing list of ingredients. After the capsules were made using the new formula, each employee was issued a bottle of "employee multi-vitamins," including a high-level employee, the Chairman of the Board. Shortly thereafter, our Chairman of the Board (a man who would naturally be very knowledgeable about pharmaceutical and nutritional products because of having the responsibility of heading up a global multi-million dollar pharmaceutical/ nutritional corporation), called the Human Resources Director to ask why the employee multi-vitamin capsules no longer included minerals. Subsequently, he educated the HR Director to the fact that vitamins cannot be readily absorbed into the body without minerals. We need minerals to absorb our vitamins.

Life is ironic - here, the company had entrusted a degreed nutritionist to reformulate our long-standing multi-vitamin product, and the nutritionist must not have known that minerals were needed in our product to make it "effective." The point I would like to re-emphasize here is there are likely many nutritional products on the market which are not going to be effective because they were never proven to be effective by means of a human clinical trial. A nutritional product might have been formulated by someone who believes he or she put an effective nutritional formula together, when that might not be the case. And, once you consume nutritional products that have not been proven effective by means of a human clinical trial, the only benefit you may end up receiving (other than potentially a placebo benefit), is, as the old saying goes, that you will have "very expensive urine."

MARKETING TACTICS

Also, when comparing products, remember that marketers can be very clever with statistics and numbers. For example, if they are claiming a percentage increase in Adult Stem Cell count, determine if the percentage increase the company is claiming occurred either as a result of a cumulative effect over a number of days or even weeks, or if the percentage increase in Adult Stem Cell count occurred in only a matter of a few hours. A 25% increase in an Adult Stem Cell count in a human within one hour of consumption would be much more significant than a 70% cumulative increase in an Adult Stem Cell count over a period of two weeks in a Petri dish. So, it is not always the highest advertised number that you should focus on; marketing professionals know how to manipulate statistics to get you to buy their products. Do your homework, including the math, and determine for yourself which product would provide you the best value for your hard earned money.

RESULTS REPORTED BY THOSE TAKING ADULT STEM CELL ENHANCER CAPSULES

Dr. Vic and I would like to share with you that we personally know at least 20 different people who are taking the same Adult Stem Cell enhancer capsules we are taking (the same nutritional capsules that influenced my Adult Stem Cells to restore my original hair color). The personal testimonies we have heard from those people are varied and many of their testimonies would likely amaze you. People have told us that as a result of taking the capsules, they have noticed improvements in a multitude of areas.

Personal Story of Victor Neugebauer, M.D. RET. now age 77:

I have experienced about ten different improvements since I started taking the Adult Stem Cell enhancer nutritional capsules 1.5 years ago. I had been deteriorating a great more than I realized as evidenced by the following improvements:

1. The two leg ulcers on both lower legs near my ankles I previously had went away within 3 to 4 weeks and have never recurred.
2. I had developed a large raised, crusted skin lesion covering nearly the entire back of my right forearm with other smaller areas showing up on the other arm, body, and legs. My skin

problems have been slowly resolving, the small areas on other areas of my body are gone and the large area on the back of my right forearm is at least 95% cleared and continues to slowly improve.

3. Several skin tags have gone away.
4. Almost all of my scars (mostly surgical) have either gone away completely or become non-raised thin white lines.
5. My gray, pasty skin complexion reverted to a healthy looking normal light brown in 2 weeks.
6. I had a somewhat problematic situation with my left knee from an automobile accident which resulted in a medial meniscus cartilage removal 50 years ago. There is absolutely no discomfort or tenderness at all in the knee now.
7. I had a gray film over my eyes which went away within 2 weeks. My vision has improved considerably and my visual correction has even reverted to what it was when I was much younger. I suspect that I had developed cataracts, which likely have been at least partially repaired by my Adult Stem Cells.
8. I was nearly bald with just a rim of gray hair around the top of my head. I have grown back a lot of hair on the top of my head and brown hair now shows on my head and beard. My body hair is now almost all brown.
9. I seem to be getting a more restful sleep, because I do not seem to require as much sleep as I used to, and I seem to remember more of my dreams.
10. My memory and my mental function seem to be constantly improving.

Now, please realize that the Adult Stem Cell enhancer nutritional capsules I have been taking are dietary supplements and they are not intended to diagnose, treat, prevent or mitigate any disease. With this F.D.A. required disclaimer done, let me say this: This product did absolutely nothing for any of my health problems. The nutritional capsules only increased moderately the level of Adult Stem Cells circulating in my blood for a few hours at a time. Those increased number of Adult Stem Cells were likely responsible for replacing, repairing, and regenerating dead and damaged cells throughout my body. Adult Stem Cells normally and naturally do this, though this activity (Adult Stem Cell repair) is greatly reduced as we age.

In conclusion, all of the above changes that are visible have been observed and commented on by my friends who have known me for years or are members of my Adult Stem Cell Advocate group. I just feel better and younger with more strength and endurance. As of this writing, I just turned 77 years of age, and as I tell my friends and other acquaintances, I feel 50 to 55 years old. I jokingly tell everyone that I intend to remain a charter member of my own personal 4-H club - that is Healthy, Happy, Horny, and Holistic, until the day I die, and I want everyone else to also stay a member.

If Dr. Vic and I took all the people that we have introduced the Adult Stem Cell enhancer nutritional capsules to and developed a list documenting all their reported improvements, it would probably warm your heart and possibly bring tears to your eyes if you contemplated how much better these people are feeling now compared to before. But, we shouldn't be

surprised at all these people's amazing results because Adult Stem Cells are so incredible.

At least three people I introduced the Adult Stem Cell enhancer capsules to have thanked me "for giving them their life back." As I already mentioned, the baby boomers and seniors are getting the most noticeable results. This is likely because older people normally have fewer Adult Stem Cells in circulation when compared to younger people.

YOUNGER PEOPLE GETTING RESULTS TOO

Younger people are also experiencing great results. I received an e-mail from a lady 30 years of age thanking me for introducing the Adult Stem Cell enhancer capsules to her. She wrote me the following: "Within three days of taking the Adult Stem Cell enhancer capsules, I felt a change and I grew in confidence as I started to feel better. The change in me is nothing short of astonishing." She then continued her e-mail writing: "While I give all the glory to Jesus Christ for this change, I do firmly believe that He is using the Adult Stem Cell enhancer capsules to play a major role in my rejuvenation. I feel like I've been given a second chance at life."
E-mail sent from Ami M. – Detroit Metro area

BOOSTING STEM CELL COUNT ENHANCES ATHLETIC PROWESS

You may find it interesting to know that on July 27, 2010, the *Wall Street Journal* ran an article entitled, "When Milliseconds Mean Everything," about riders in the Tour de France. In that article, it was reported that one of the team doctors, Dr. Van Bommel, relayed his "favorite new idea: an algae-based product that triggers the release of more Stem Cells from the bone marrow into the blood stream." So apparently, even some of the cyclists in the Tour de France are aware of the benefits of boosting their Adult Stem Cell count (with an all-natural product) for increased energy. (Miller, 2010, para. 12)

ADULT STEM CELL ENHANCERS COMPARED TO NUTRITIONAL SUPPLEMENTS AND RX DRUGS

When we take Adult Stem Cell enhancers to increase the number of Adult Stem Cells in our blood circulation, this will yield a much different result than taking ordinary nutritional supplements or over-the-counter (OTC) or prescription drugs. **Why? Adult Stem Cell enhancers just don't nourish cells like many other types of nutritional supplements do or suppress situations to help make us feel better like many OTC or Rx products do. Instead, by taking Adult Stem Cell enhancers, we can experience an increased number of Adult Stem Cells in our blood circulation. These extra Adult Stem Cells can actually help repair and reverse the situations from which we have been suffering.**

Wouldn't you rather reverse your situations, rather than continue to live with those problems? Please re-read the bold underlined information in the above paragraph several times until you firmly grasp the significance of the amazing power and anti-aging potential of your own Adult Stem Cells. Because once you process and understand that vital information and take steps to increase your Adult Stem Cell count, you will greatly enhance your chances of anti-aging and achieving optimal wellness.

As mentioned earlier in this book, in addition to Adult Stem Cells having the ability to repair most (if not "ALL") situations in your body, Adult Stem Cells have the innate intelligence to know what to repair first in order of importance. As Victor Neugebauer, M.D. RET. relays: "First they (Adult Stem Cells) will fix the life threatening situations, before they will fix the comfort situations."

For example, let's say that you had terrible hip discomfort and also a liver situation, as a result of your liver breaking down. Because your hip is causing you so much discomfort, you might strongly desire that your Adult Stem Cells would fix your hip situation in quick order. But, your hip problem is not a life threatening situation – it may be tremendously uncomfortable, but you will not die from having hip discomfort. Instead, with your hypothetical liver situation, and your Adult Stem Cells having the innate intelligence to know what to fix first in order of importance, your Adult Stem Cells will initially work to resolve your liver situation (a life supporting organ), before your Adult Stem Cells will begin to fix your hip situation.

Note: By now you should realize that by increasing your Adult Stem Cell count, your body can start regenerating itself. As your body begins the repair process, your bodily changes could include re-growing nerves, capillaries or blood vessels. As a consequence, you might start feeling sensations similar to when you were a child, which your mother would call "growing pains." Do not let those sensations scare or discourage you from continuing to take Adult Stem Cell enhancer capsules (or undergoing Adult Stem Cell Therapy). Welcome those new sensations as your body starts

taking steps to repair itself with an increased Adult
Stem Cell count.

ADULT STEM CELL ENHANCERS FOR PETS
The Adult Stem Cell enhancer product we are taking is
also available in a modified version for pets as a liver-
flavor chewable tablet. Actually, one of the ladies who
introduced us to the Adult Stem Cell enhancer
nutritional capsules initially learned about the capsules
as a result of giving the liver flavor chewable tablets to
her dog. She was so impressed with the results her dog
experienced from the chewable version that she
telephoned the women who sold her the pet version of
the product, and said to her, "After two weeks of
giving the chewable tablets to our dog, with such a
marked improvement in how our dog walks, we know
that it works amazingly well on dogs. Do you happen to
know if the company making the pet product also
makes an Adult Stem Cell enhancer product for
people?" The lady who sold her the chewable tablets
replied, "Of course the company does, the Adult Stem
Cell enhancer pet product I sold you was originally
formulated for people. Because there were so many
people getting such great results, the company decided
to develop a pet version of the product; and, as you
saw with your dog, the pet product works wonderfully
well, too."

I know several people who have given the chewable
Adult Stem Cell enhancers to their dogs. The reported
benefits their pets received follow:

1. One lady I know began giving her daughter's 13-
   year-old Cocker Spaniel the Adult Stem Cell
   enhancers and "within two weeks of putting the

dog on the product, she said the dog started running around like a puppy."

2. A man I know began giving the Adult Stem Cell enhancer capsules to his 11-year-old Sheltie and within 3 weeks, he noticed that his Sheltie always appeared like it just had a bath because the Sheltie's coat started looking so shiny.

The Adult Stem Cell enhancer product we take is also available in pellet form for horses. So, even the pets we love can experience benefits from taking an Adult Stem Cell enhancer.

NUTRIENTS TO HELP ADULT STEM CELLS
To help ensure our Adult Stem Cells will be able reach the organs and tissues that need repairing, Dr. Vic and I are also taking another nutritional product that contains enzymes known for their ability to dissolve excess fibrin in blood. Many people over age 50 have too much fibrin in their blood. The older we are, the more fibrin we have. Fibrin has been described to me as almost like "a netting or mesh" in our blood. (A Phlebotomist - a person who takes blood samples from people's veins - said to me that she doesn't know how some older people's blood can even flow through their veins because she has seen how thick their blood looks with excess fibrin.) Too much fibrin in our blood can prevent our Adult Stem Cells from getting into our capillaries, making them unable to reach their target. So, if you are over age 50, taking an enzyme known to dissolve excess fibrin is something you should consider. And/or, to improve your blood circulation, thus increasing your chances that your Adult Stem Cells will be able to reach areas of distress, you may want to

consider supplementing your diet with a mushroom revered by the Chinese for over 4,000 years called Ganoderma, also known as Reishi or Lingzhi. The Ganoderma (Reishi) mushroom is also known for being very effective for detoxifying the liver. I drink a healthy coffee every day that is infused with the Ganoderma (Reishi) mushroom. Research Ganoderma or Reishi yourself on the Internet, and you would probably be amazed to learn why the Chinese have revered this very special mushroom for thousands of years.

And, of course it goes without saying, with most of us being on the Standard American Diet, we should all consider supplementing our diet with good quality nutritional products each day, including the essential B Vitamins, Vitamin D3, Vitamin C and Omega3. Eat plenty of fresh fruits and vegetables (organic whenever possible). The earth supplies us with whole foods to keep us healthy, not processed chemical-laden foods. Also, be sure to drink plenty of filtered water and green tea (green tea is noted to enhance Adult Stem Cell proliferation).

Further, if you are a smoker, think seriously about quitting the habit, because studies show the effects of smoking can seriously impede Adult Stem Cells.

BREAK OPEN YOUR "PIGGY BANK" AND GIVE IT A TRY
If you have not taken an Adult Stem Cell enhancer before, you owe it to yourself to consider "opening up your purse strings." In terms of anti-aging, if you take an Adult Stem Cell enhancer that has been proven effective in a human clinical trial, you should get a tremendous "bang for your buck." There are thousands

of nutritional supplements on the market that can nourish your cells, but only a nutritional supplement that leads to an increased Adult Stem Cell count will give your body what it needs to potentially regenerate itself. If you take that leap of faith and start taking an Adult Stem Cell enhancer, you should make the commitment to take it for at least six months to assess your results and give your body time to repair. Remember, your Adult Stem Cells go to the areas most in need of repair first, and if that happens to be your organs, you may not feel any difference at all as your organs are being slowly repaired. Rome was not built in a day. It took you many years to get your body in this aged condition, so it may take anywhere from several days to many months before you start noticing any positive effects from taking an Adult Stem Cell enhancer. If you take steps to continue to educate yourself about Adult Stem Cells, you will come to realize that regardless of whether or not you actually notice any bodily changes from taking an Adult Stem Cell enhancer (which has been proven effective in a Human Clinical Trial), your body is still benefiting by having an increased Adult Stem Cell count.

Also, if you begin taking an Adult Stem Cell enhancer, start out slowly (such as taking only one-half the recommended daily amount appearing on the product label) for the first several weeks. Give your body time to adjust. If you do not start out slowly, your body may experience some unfavorable situations as your increased amount of Adult Stem Cells go to work to naturally repair and detoxify your body. Those situations could include stomach discomfort, etc. Read the product label carefully before starting the product.

Some people have told me that even though they are spending money on the Adult Stem Cell enhancer nutritional capsules we are taking, they have been able to reduce other expenditures. Why would that be the case? For example, with an increased Adult Stem Cell count (resulting from taking the nutritional capsules) some people might experience their fingernails becoming harder, so they may no longer feel it necessary to continue to go to the nail salon to get acrylic nails. Or, as another example, some people may no longer feel they need to spend money on hair dyes. And, of course it goes without saying that someone who is in better condition as a result of an increased Adult Stem Cell count will very likely not need to spend as much money on bodily repairs, so to speak.

Remember, Adult Stem Cell enhancers do <u>not</u> fix or repair anything in your body. Adult Stem Cell enhancers simply influence your bone marrow to release extra Adult Stem Cells. Once those extra Adult Stem Cells are in your blood circulation, with their ability to change to become any type of specialized cell in your body, they seek out areas of distress for restorative and anti-aging purposes.

<u>IF YOU WANT MORE INFORMATION ABOUT AN ADULT STEM CELL ENHANCER:</u>

Note: As mentioned earlier in this book, we have not shared with you the brand name of the Adult Stem Cell enhancer nutritional capsules we are taking. That is because t**he purpose of this book is to educate people about the anti-aging abilities of Adult Stem Cells** and **some steps people can take to increase their Adult**

Stem Cell count, <u>NOT</u> to sell Adult Stem Cell enhancer capsules. However, after you finish reading our book, if you decide that you want more information or the brand name of the Adult Stem Cell enhancer capsules we take, which were <u>proven effective in a human clinical trial</u>, feel free to access your co-authors' website at: <u>www.therealnewfountainofyouth.com</u> to learn more. (Also, our contact information appears in the front of our book.) Or, if someone recommended this book to you, check with that person because that individual may already be taking an Adult Stem Cell enhancer.

CHAPTER 5 – (EXERCISE CAN INCREASE ADULT STEM CELL COUNT)

<u>CLINICAL TRIAL RESULTS CONCERNING EXERCISE</u>
On December 26, 2012, the *World Journal of Cardiology* published a study entitled, "Circulating endothelial and progenitor cells: Evidence from acute and long-term exercise effects." The conclusions of the study were "<u>that physical activity, either performed as a single exercise session or performed as part of an exercise training program, resulted in a significant increase in circulating bone marrow derived cells</u> (Endothelial Progenitor Cells)." ("Circulating endothelial and progenitor cells: Evidence from acute and long-term exercise effects," 2012, p. 324).

Also, as proven in a clinical study with the participants being rats: "Professor Dafna Benayahu and her scientific research team had rats run on a treadmill device 20 minutes a day for 13 weeks (obviously an intensive and consistent form of exercise for a rat to run 20 minutes per day for 13 weeks). At the end of the 13 week study, conducted at Tel Aviv University's Sackler School of Medicine, <u>results showed that the average Stem Cell count of the rats had increased by over 20%.</u>"   (Senior Journal, 2010, para. 7)

<u>THINK ABOUT EXERCISE</u>
Ever wonder why people who exercise on a consistent basis often appear younger looking than others you know who are more sedentary?   (Adult Stem Cells can repair wrinkles, too.)   As shown in the clinical studies mentioned above, exercise can increase our Adult Stem Cell count. Or, do you ever wonder why so many young children are now developing diabetes?   We keep hearing in the news that there is a "diabetic epidemic" and how children now are commonly experiencing "adult onset (type II) diabetes."   Prior to fifteen or so years ago, this was not the case. However, today in our technically advanced society, most children rarely exercise, preferring to stay "glued" to their computers, cell-phones, electronic games, or televisions.

<u>THE DOWNSIDE OF LIVING IN THE TECHNO WORLD</u>
With this "technology addiction," it is becoming quite rare for children to want to go outside to play with their friends because children know the time spent exercising would result in being disconnected from the "techno world."   Do you know that in several countries in the orient, parents are now sending their children to rehabilitation classes in the hopes their children will learn how to recover from their "technology addiction?"   Why?   Because, children do not want to disengage themselves from their computers.   It has been reported in the media that in some oriental countries, several children have died as a result of

sitting at their computer for more than 50 hours straight playing techno games.

As you may be aware, diabetes (whether it is being experienced by adults or children) occurs when our pancreas breaks down. Wouldn't it make sense that if we had enough Adult Stem Cells in blood circulation that an adequate supply of Adult Stem Cells could work to repair our pancreas to keep it optimally functioning?

Exciting news for those with type I diabetes: As revealed on January 12, 2012, in *Medical News Today*, – "Stem Cells from (umbilical and placenta) cord blood "re-educated" the immune system "T Cells" of people with type 1 diabetes so their pancreas started producing insulin again, thereby reducing the amount of insulin they needed to inject. The results showed the median daily dose of required insulin was down by 38% at week 12 for the six patients with moderate diabetes and by 25% for the patients with severe diabetes. There was no change in required insulin dose for the controls. These were the findings of a study led by Dr Yong Zhao, from University of Illinois at Chicago." (Paddock, Ph.D., 2012, para. 1, 9)

My (Ann's) father developed type II diabetes when he was in his early sixties. After he was diagnosed with diabetes, he was required to take insulin shots. Shortly thereafter, he began a regular exercise program. With regular exercise, his insulin levels improved so much that he no longer needed to take insulin shots; instead, he only took insulin in pill form. Then, twenty years later, at age 83, after having a stroke, he stopped exercising altogether. Soon thereafter, his insulin levels got worse and he was again required to take insulin shots.   Knowing that exercise can increase an Adult Stem Cell count, I suspect that during the 20+ years he was regularly exercising, his Adult Stem Cell count was high enough to keep the pancreas functioning fairly well.   Then, when he stopped exercising, his circulating Adult Stem Cells naturally declined (as a result of lack of exercise), which adversely affected his pancreas.

So, do whatever you can to influence your grandchildren (or children) to disengage them from the "techno world" and to take time to exercise each day. Such exercise will help safeguard their well being and increase their Adult Stem Cell count.

Start getting serious about exercising yourself to achieve optimal health and increase your own Adult Stem Cell count.   Before you begin an exercise program, remember to consult your physician to get advice about what exercise program is recommended for you.

GET INSPIRED TO EXERCISE
As a result of reading an exceptional book entitled *Younger Next Year* for Women* by Chris Crowley and Harry S. Lodge, M.D. (originally published as *Younger Next Year* (for men), I was "scared straight" about the importance of exercise, and I now appreciate the value of exercising every day.   The authors of that book relayed they believe within the next 20 years, experts will determine that not exercising will be as harmful to the body as smoking two packs of cigarettes – now that statement helped to scare me enough to realize I better not miss a day of exercise. (Crowley, Lodge, M.D., 2005, p. 59) After finishing that book, I believe

everyone should make exercise a number one priority each day. The authors of *Younger Next Year* recommend people should view exercise as seriously as the commitment of going to work every day; and also a person's planned exercise routine should be performed the same time every day. For me, if I do my exercise routine first thing in the morning, then all the other things for which I am responsible will not get in the way. I hope you read *Younger Next Year*. If you read that book, it may turn out to be one of the most inspiring books you have ever read. Coincidentally, after I started reading the version for women, Dan B., a fellow residing in southeast Michigan, told me that he had read *Younger Next Year* (for men) three times. He said the book had such a positive influence on him, that following the advice of the authors, he lost over 40 pounds in one year's time, and now, he fully intends to lose another 30 pounds by continuing his daily exercise regime. Also, a woman I know read *Younger Next Year* for Women* and found it so inspiring that she later purchased additional copies for each of her three daughters.

Here is another reason to exercise: "Based on the results of a 10 year study of 1,765 participants, if you are fit in mid-life, you **double** your chance of surviving to 85..... Put another way: If you're not fit in your 50s, your projected life span is eight years shorter than if you are fit. Fitness even trumped smoking cessation in the magnitude of benefit among participants in the study." (Winslow, 2010)

One more reason to exercise – brain function: You've probably already heard that exercise is also good for your brain function. Why? Per Jack Kessler, M.D.,

Chairman of Neurology at Northwestern University's School of Medicine in Chicago, "Your brain is packed with Adult Stem Cells. As we age, these Stem Cells tend to become less responsive. They don't divide as readily and can slump into a kind of cellular sleep. Adult Stem Cells have the capacity to divide into new Stem Cells or into new neurons. Exercise helps to ensure that neuronal Stem Cells stay lively and new brain cells are born." (Reynolds 2010, para. 3)

Many baby boomers and seniors are not as active as they were when they were younger. As exercise has been shown to increase Adult Stem Cells in blood circulation, doesn't it make sense that baby boomers and seniors (who tend not to exercise as much as when they were younger) would have far less Adult Stem Cells in circulation than younger people do?

GET INSPIRED TO EXERCISE WITH MUSIC
As a result of reading *Younger Next Year* for Women, I made a resolution to take a 20-30 minute brisk walk every day.   To help my walks seem more enjoyable, I often listen to music on my IPod including songs written by my favorite musician/composer, Al Conway. Al is an extremely talented artist and composer, and he composes much of his music while travelling to different parts of the world. He has composed works in spectacular locations such as the Swiss Alps; Norwegian Fjords; Cook's Bay, Tahiti; Glacier National Park, and many other locations across the globe.   With him recognizing that many people like to listen to music while they exercise and also being aware that exercise is very beneficial to Adult Stem Cell proliferation, he put together a collection of some of his upbeat music which he has entitled: *THE NEW FOUNTAIN OF YOUTH*

– MUSIC YOU NEED NOW. If you are serious about exercising while listening to music, with a possible interest in learning how you could obtain Al Conway's upbeat *NEW FOUNTAIN OF YOUTH – MUSIC YOU NEED NOW* song collection, feel free to access our website at: www.therealnewfountainofyouth.com. If you have ever listened to music with the intention of brightening up your day, chances are you would highly enjoy listening to Al Conway's music when you exercise to increase your Adult Stem Cell count.

Now, some of you may feel that you are unable to exercise because of your current physical condition. Perhaps some people reading this book are confined to a wheelchair or significantly over-weight. We are all different. So, for those who believe they are unable to exercise or who are considerably "out-of-shape," I recommend you consider searching the Internet for an exercise program called "Flip Fitness." The program consists of a deck of instructional cards developed by a lady who wanted to inspire her invalid mother to exercise. Using the "Flip Fitness" cards as a reference, you can build your strength and endurance, while having some fun at the same time. I learned about "Flip Fitness" from Bob G., a fellow living in Arizona, who told me he significantly improved his physical stamina because the "Flip Fitness Program" continually motivated him to strive to reach a higher fitness level. http//flipfitness.com

Make sure you get plenty of exercise each day to help increase your Adult Stem Cell count to an optimal level. And, for anti-aging purposes, exercise is probably the most economical way to increase your Adult Stem Cell count.

CHAPTER 6 – (COLD LIGHT LEVEL LASERS CAN AFFECT ADULT STEM CELLS)

COLD LIGHT LASERS LEAD TO STEM CELL PROLIFERATION

As we previously mentioned early on in this book, in conjunction with Stem Cell Therapy, cold light level lasers are frequently used to re-activate Stem Cells before, and sometimes even after, the Adult Stem Cells are injected into people.

INCREASE YOUR STEM CELL COUNT WITH A HAND HELD DEVICE (the size of a remote control for your T.V. set) USING A "COLD LIGHT LEVEL LASER"

Cold light level lasers, otherwise known as low light level lasers or soft lasers, emit warm light that can help to increase blood circulation. I (Ann) own an F.D.A. registered cold light level laser for over-the-counter (OTC) home use. It is about the size of a remote control for my television set, and it fits nicely in the palm of my hand. Many of you have heard of hot lasers, the lasers surgeons use as cutting devices during surgery. But, I am not talking about those types of lasers. I am talking about a cold light level laser. As contrasted to the lasers surgeons use, cold light level lasers emit warm, gentle light. Many massage therapists, veterinarians, dentists, and chiropractors now use cold light level lasers in their spas and clinics to expedite the recovery process. For cosmetic purposes, cold light level lasers are being used by people to re-grow hair and enhance collagen. Also, chances are if you opt to have Stem Cell Therapy the utilization of a cold light level laser will probably be integrated into your treatment.

About 40 years ago, scientists discovered the benefits of cold light level lasers. In the United States, the F.D.A. approved cold light level lasers for human use in the year 2000; and in 2005, the F.D.A. started approving some cold light level lasers for over-the-counter use.

With the dozens of hours I have spent conducting Internet research about cold light level lasers, and having attended many laser seminars, I am well versed on the subject of cold light level lasers.

One of the most important benefits of cold light level lasers is they emit coherent light in the form of photons. Photons are used by the mitochondria of our cells to stimulate ATP (Adenosine Triphosphate) production in our cells, which in turn, provides the energy our cells need to optimally perform their many cellular functions. Similar to how the cells of plants use photons from the sun to grow, photons donated by cold lasers enter our body's cells to help grow and energize our cells.

Ever wonder how our esteemed athletes can rebound much quicker from their injuries compared to many years ago? Years ago, injured athletes were frequently out for the entire season. Today, oftentimes our esteemed athletes "are back in play" in only a matter of a few weeks. That is because many of these athletes are getting cold light level laser treatments to facilitate their recoveries.

The cold light level laser device I own is registered with the F.D.A. for "pain, inflammation, circulation, relaxation and arthritis." Now, if you could get benefits in all those five different areas from using a cold light level laser, and with the predicted life of the laser I own being about ten years, wouldn't you think you (and your family and also your pets) could get a favorable return on your investment if you were to purchase a comparable laser? Think about it, is there any other household appliance you own that has a predicted operating life of ten years?

Nicely enough, the laser I own is made in the "good old U.S.A." So, with me believing that many products being made in the United States are of a higher quality, I feel confident that, with the ten year predicted life of my cold light level laser, I will be getting many years of good use from it and realize an excellent return on investment.

I would not want to part with my laser for "all the tea in China." I love my laser, and I strongly believe every household in America should own a comparable laser to the one I own for the benefit of themselves, their family, and their pets.

If you would like to learn more about the benefits of cold light level lasers and how they can positively influence the cells in your body, you may want to consider reading an interesting and informative book entitled *Stillpoint Laser - Unwind and Dissolve Into Your Quantumfield* by Paul and Lillie Weisbart.

NOTE: Please be aware that if you purchase or use a cold light level laser, you make sure you read the safety precautions. Check with a medical professional about using a cold light level laser. Unlike the laser I own, many cold light level lasers on the market emit a beam of light that, without taking appropriate protective measures could possibly cause damage to people's eyes. Also, if you start using a cold light level laser, do a skin test first because there are some people who have skin sensitivities to cold light level lasers. If you begin to research the topic of cold light level lasers further, you will learn that one of the biggest challenges in getting the best results is determining the "ideal length of time" to shine a laser over an area. Scientists and medical doctors have found in clinical trials that it is difficult to determine the ideal "exposure time," and they recognize that they need to also take into account "the bell shape curve," as it relates to the possibility of "diminishing returns."

PROFESSOR DEMONSTRATES EFFECTIVENESS OF COLD LIGHT LEVEL LASER ON ADULT STEM CELLS:

In August 2011, Professor Uri Oron, in Tel Aviv, with his background in lasers, made an amazing discovery. Because he was aware cold light level lasers were being used to re-activate Stem Cells in—vitro (outside the body), he suspected cold light level lasers could stimulate Adult Stem Cells in-vivo (inside the body) "using a non-invasive approach." He, along with his scientific team, demonstrated that his theory was correct by shining a cold light level laser "into (over) a heart attack victim's bone marrow. Consequently, the heart attack victim had an 80% reduction in the formation of scar tissue around the site of the damaged heart. Thereafter, the Professor and his team of scientists also demonstrated the same effect could be achieved by shining a cold light level laser into (over) the bone marrow of animals after the animals had experienced a heart attack. Why did these heart attack victims in the study (animals and one human) have as much as an 80% reduction in the scarring of their hearts after they sustained their heart attacks? Professor Oron theorizes: "After we stimulate the cells with the laser and enhance their proliferation in the bone marrow, it's likely that more cells migrate into the bloodstream. The cells that eventually reach the heart secrete growth factors to a higher extent, and new blood vessel formation is encouraged." (ScienceDaily, 2011)

At this point in the book, we should have all come to the realization that Adult Stem Cells can regenerate organs and tissues. Knowing this, coupled with Professor Oron's discovery, I make sure I regularly shine my cold light level laser over my own bone marrow to increase my Adult Stem Cell count. With me already possessing a cold light level laser in my household, other than the cost of the electricity used to charge my laser's battery, it costs me absolutely nothing, except my time, to potentially increase my Adult Stem Cell count by shining my cold light level laser over my bone marrow.

Being aware that shining a cold light level laser over bone marrow has the potential to significantly reduce scarring after a heart attack occurs, most anyone would have adequate justification to purchase a cold light level laser as a proactive measure. If you were to take the time to investigate the subject of cold light level lasers, you would come to realize a versatile cold light level laser like I own can serve as a form of an extra insurance policy, somewhat equivalent to a high-tech first-aid kit.

REV UP YOUR ADULT STEM CELL POWER –
YOU NEED IT NOW!

ADULT STEM CELLS FROM RED BONE MARROW

When we talk about Adult Stem Cells coming out of our bone marrow, we are talking about red bone marrow, not yellow bone marrow. I have read that as children, we have a lot more red bone marrow compared to adults. When we are young and our are growing, we have more Adult Stem Cells in circulation and more red bone marrow than adults do. Then, after we are grown, as a part of our aging process, our red bone marrow in our long bones (in our arms and legs), converts to yellow bone marrow. So, in adults, red bone marrow is most commonly found in places like our pelvic bones, hip bones, our ribs and our skull. Having this knowledge, I now make it a point to shine my cold light level laser device over some of the aforementioned areas several times per week to potentially increase in my Adult Stem Cell count.

Remember, cold light level lasers donate photons, which Professor Oron and his scientific team theorize influences our bone marrow to release extra Adult Stem Cells. Once those extra Adult Stem Cells are in our blood circulation, they seek out organs and tissues in distress for purposes of repair and anti-aging.

AFTERWORD

BEWARE OF SCARE TACTICS

Before closing this book, please remember that just as there are people working in the oil industry who would not want us to use alternative fuels, there are people in other industries who have vested interests, too. So, I would like to mention that there are some people working in various organizations and professions whose economic interests could be adversely affected as the role of Adult Stem Cells becomes more widely known. Some of these people have very strong influences over the news media and a presence on the Internet and are working very hard to effectively scare you from looking into anything related to Adult Stem Cells. For that reason, you may see only a smattering of information appearing in the news media about Adult Stem Cells. Conversely, you may see things in the media or on the Internet that attempt to make you afraid of Adult Stem Cells, Adult Stem Cell related products, and Adult Stem Cell Therapies.

Do not be afraid of your Adult Stem Cells and their amazing powers. As previously mentioned, Adult Stem Cells were responsible for growing your body, and they are keeping you alive. Your bone marrow makes significant numbers of Adult Stem Cells every day for the purpose of improving your overall health, and in great enough numbers in blood circulation, your Adult Stem Cells have the potential to rejuvenate and anti-age you. Embrace your Adult Stem Cells, and do what it takes to benefit the most from this newly discovered "Fountain of Youth."

As we near the "home stretch," let us summarize the high points in this book:

The amazing power of Adult Stem Cells was revealed in the beginning of the 21st Century, when scientists discovered that Adult Stem Cells enter our blood circulation to seek out areas of distress. Once our Adult Stem Cells reach those areas of distress, they have the potential to become any type of specialized cell in our bodies including brain cells, heart cells, liver cells, etc. The role of Adult Stem Cells is to regenerate our bodies. A high Adult Stem Cell count has the potential to slow down and even reverse our aging process. Adult Stem Cells are part of our Natural Renewal System; they function as a built-in repair kit, and they are our internal "Fountain of Youth."

Until the year 2000, never in the recorded history of mankind was the true versatility of Adult Stem Cells known. All of us are very fortunate to be living in today's time. Your grandparents and maybe even your parents, had to suffer from physical and psychological situations for which you may now be able to avoid simply by harnessing the incredible power of your Adult Stem Cells and taking steps to "rev up" your Adult Stem Cell count. Our hope for you baby boomers, seniors, and all others who have the desire to anti-age is that you grasp the significance of the amazing and miraculous power of your Adult Stem Cells and you take steps to enhance their abilities.

Remember what Leo Feocht, M.D., and William Hoffman were quoted as saying in the January 12, 2012, edition of *the Atlantic* magazine, "Stem Cells are proving to be the silver bullet, and the Holy Grail....They could alleviate ALL manner of suffering, whether it's caused by disease, injury or genetic fate...they have the power to regenerate tissue that is healthy and repair tissue that is diseased or damaged." (Furtch/Hoffman, 2012, para. 7)

Remember Roger Nocera, M.D., who relayed in his book, *Cells That Heal Us From Cradle To Grave*, that a high Adult Stem Cell count can curtail atherosclerosis and assist in the neurological recovery after a stroke. (Nocera, M.D., 2011, p. 38 and p. 41)

REV UP YOUR ADULT STEM CELL POWER –
YOU NEED IT NOW!

Remember that it was shown by an animal clinical trial that muscle Stem Cells are increased as a result of regular intensive exercise. (Senior Journal, 2010, para. 2)

Remember Professor Oron's discovery that shining a cold light level laser into (over) the bone marrow can significantly reduce the amount of scarring after a heart attack occurs, which he theorizes is a result of enhanced Adult Stem Cell proliferation. (ScienceDaily, 2011)

Oh, and I almost forgot to mention, in case you are wondering if Ruby, my friend who has been an entertainer for 30+ years, ever noticed any results after she started taking the Adult Stem Cell enhancer capsules. Well, of course, she did. Soon after Ruby started taking the capsules, she felt so much more energy that she felt inspired to repaint every room in her home. Then, she installed all new flooring throughout and redecorated each room with completely new (or gently used) furniture, wall paintings, knick-knacks, etc. Also, as you may recall, before she began taking the Adult Stem Cell enhancer nutritional capsules, all she could do was to talk about retiring from show business. Since then, all she talks about is wanting to take on as many new "gigs" as she can handle. Yes, like many other baby boomers, including myself, Ruby is another person who has experienced "new found energy" and is also looking younger as a result of having an increased Adult Stem Cell count. Like my husband, Dr. Vic, and many of my friends, Ruby would not want to go a day without taking her Adult Stem Cell enhancer capsules.

As for myself, with the scientific knowledge I have acquired on the subject of Adult Stem Cells, I feel confident that each day I work to increase my Adult Stem Cell count with the methods Dr. Vic and I have described to you in this book, that I am getting younger every day. It is my theory that every day I take steps to increase my Adult Stem Cell count, my body is getting one day younger, and for those who are not taking those steps their bodies are getting one day older. (Remember *Merriam-Webster's* definition of aging we mentioned early on in our book?) Please note that I have observed the faces of my friends who are working to increase their Adult Stem Cell count, and I am amazed at how much younger their faces look when I periodically meet up with them. Changes to my friends' faces have included having rosier cheeks, looking less pale, and even looking more alert. To further back my theory, consider what Professor Dafna Benayahu and her team at Tel Aviv University's Sackler School of Medicine say, "Exercise unlocks the Stem Cells of our muscles, and exercise makes us look younger." (Senior Journal, 2010, para. 2)

Remember, as previously mentioned, our Adult Stem Cells will have a much better chance of getting to areas of bodily distress if we take steps to detoxify our body of heavy metals and also take specific enzymes to reduce the amount of fibrin in our blood.

So, what have you done today to optimize you Adult Stem Cell System's anti-aging potential so you too can experience the miraculous benefits of the newly discovered "Fountain of Youth?" **It's easy as 1-2-3:**

1. Take an Adult Stem Cell enhancer (Preferably, an Adult Stem Cell enhancer which has been proven in a <u>human clinical trial</u> to significantly increase Adult Stem Cells in blood circulation.) Read the product label carefully before starting the product.
2. Get plenty of regular daily exercise. (Remember to consult your physician for approval.)
3. Shine an F.D.A. registered OTC cold light level laser over your red bone marrow (Reminder: Remember, for us adults, red bone marrow is located in our hips, pelvic bone, ribs, and skull.) USE PROPER SAFETY PRECAUTIONS WITH LASERS.

Or, if you decide to take Adult Stem Cell Therapy, which can dramatically increase your Adult Stem Cell count, you may be amazed at how quickly your organs and tissues renew, repair and regenerate. There are now tens of thousands (maybe even hundreds of thousands) of people across the globe who have already taken Stem Cell Therapy, and many of those people have proclaimed exceptional results. (Remember, to ask your doctor about the possibility of any associated risks.)

Never underestimate the power of your Adult Stem Cells. Yes, we baby boomers and others who are interested in anti-aging are very fortunate to be living at the start of the "Stem Cell Age." Rest assured, with what you know now, if you take steps to increase your Adult Stem Cell count, you will have the potential to anti-age yourself, look and feel younger, and increase your chances of avoiding needless suffering while enjoying a better quality of life with your family, friends and your pets.

In the upcoming years, we anticipate that considerably more information will become known about the amazing role of Adult Stem Cells. Because of their incredible restorative and regenerative abilities, could it eventually come to pass that scientists officially rename Adult Stem Cells, "Healing Cells?" As mentioned earlier in this book, author Roger M. Nocera, M.D., and others associated with the Vatican have already been calling them just that – "Healing Cells."

In the meantime, like our friends Mario and Joanne have been doing, if you want to feel as if you have a new found purpose in life, pass along your knowledge of the amazing power of Adult Stem Cells to everyone you care about. By spreading the word about the role of Adult Stem Cells, those people who you touch with your own words may be curious enough to learn about their own anti-aging internal "Fountain of Youth" during this new era – the "Stem Cell Age."

Remember the old saying we mentioned earlier in this book: "You can lead a horse to water, but you can't make it drink (think)." Dr. Vic and I hope our book will lead a multitude of horses to water (the "New Fountain of Youth"), resulting in clear-thinking, and that all will learn to harness the full anti-aging potential of their Adult Stem Cells to go on to win the "Triple Crown." Remember to keep an open-mind.

REV UP YOUR ADULT STEM CELL POWER –
YOU NEED IT NOW!

<u>Concluding words from Victor Neugebauer, M.D. RET.:</u>
In conclusion to our book, I have already lived at least 15 years longer than I expected, so every day now is a gift. I do not care about how much longer I live, just the quality of what remaining life is ahead of me, though I would prefer my death be later rather than sooner. The only thing that is certain is that we all will die some day. It is not a question of if, but when, where, and how. Good luck, good health, and wealth to you and yours. If you have any questions feel free to contact me. There is only one of me, so I may not be able to answer immediately, but I shall make every effort to answer.

Feel free to contact either Dr. Vic or Ann through:
www.therealnewfountainofyouth.com

You can also find us both on LinkedIn with the location of Tampa/St. Petersburg/Clearwater, Florida.

You have come to the end of our book, which we hope you have enjoyed. --- Remember, at the beginning of the book on page 12, we asked you to go to the Internet to watch some on-line videos? Please, if you have not watched those videos yet, do so right now and see with your own eyes the amazing and incredible power of Adult Stem Cells at work.

Remember, revere your Adult Stem Cells – they are your life-long anti-aging best friends. With this in mind, what have you done for your Adult Stem Cells lately? ☺
===============

REFERENCES

AdistemVideos (2010, April 25). General Overview of
Adistem Technology - English_Vasilis Paspaliaris [Video
file]. Retrieved from Youtube website:
http://www.youtube.com/watch?v=zGP8hxr395M

Altrocchi, MD, P. H., Ideational Change: Why is it so
Difficult to Change?
http://www.shakespearesmonument.com/ALTROCCHI%
20IDEATIONAL%20CHANGE.pdf

Berkrot, W./Krauskopf, L. (2011, November 14). UPDATE 1-
Stem Cell therapy works in heart failure trial. *Reuters*.
Retrieved from
http://www.reuters.com/article/2011/11/14/heart-
stemcells-idUSN1E7AD11920111114

Cabot, T. (2013, March 18). Whatever Happened to Stem
Cells. *Esquire*, p. 1. http://www.esquire.com/features/stem-
cells-research-politics-0413-3

CafeMomStudies (2011, December 30). Suzanne Somers'
Stem Cell Breast Reconstruction Surgery - Episode 1 [Video
file]. Retrieved from Youtube website:
http://www.youtube.com/watch?v=xt55cTQEoHk

Caplan, Ph.D., Arnold. (October 2008). *Treatment of Human
Diseases: Cell-Based Therapies using Adult Meschenchymal
Stem Cells* [PowerPoint slides]. Retrieved from
http://www.njbiomaterials.org/NJCB_Files/File/Sympo
sium/Caplan.ppt.pdf

CBS New York, (2012, February 14). Seen at 11: Could the Next Generation Live to be 150? Experts Huge Breakthroughs in Science and Technology Could Make it a Reality. *CBS New York*. Retrieved from http://newyork.cbslocal.com/2012/02/14/could-the-next-generation-live-to-be-150/

Centenohome. (2007, August 3). What's the Difference between Embryonic and Adult Stem Cells? [Video file]. Retrieved from Youtube website: http://www.youtube.com/watch?v=WaRnVcwZ0i8

Circulating endothelial and progenitor cells: Evidence from acute and long-term exercise effects. (2012, December 26). *World Journal of Cardiology, IV*(12), 312-326. Retrieved from http://www.ncbi.nlm.nih.gov/pmc/articles/PMC3530787/

Crowley, C., & Lodge, M.D., H. S. (2005). *Younger Next Year* for Women (2nd ed..) New York, New York: Workman Publishing.

Drapeau, MSc, C. (2010). *Cracking the Stem Cell Code*. Vancouver, Washington: Sutton Hart Press LLC

www.flipfitness.com . Retrieved from http://www.flipfitness.com

Furtch, L., Hoffman, Wm., (2012, January 19). The Holy Grail of Medicine: On the Mystery and Power of Stem Cells. *the Atlantic*. Retrieved from http://www.theatlantic.com/health/archive/2012/01/the-holy-grail-of-medicine-on-the-mystery-and-power-of-stem-cells/251473/

Gupta, S., Human Stem Cells at John Hopkins: A Forty Year History. *John Hopkins Medicine*. Retrieved from http://www.hopkinsmedicine.org/stem_cell_research/cell_therapy/human_stem_cells_johns_hopkins.html

Jensen, G. S., Hart, A. N., & Zaske, L.A.M., Drapeau, C., Gupta, N., Schaeffer, D.J., Cruickshank, J.A. (2007). Mobilization of CD34+CD133+ and CD34+CD133 - Stem Cells in vivo-by consumption of an extract from Aphanizomenon flos-aqueae- related to modulation of CXCR4 expression by an L-selectin ligand?. *Cardiovascular Revascular Medicine 8*, (), 189-202. Retrieved from http://www.warrenhammer.com/storage/stem-cell/Stem-Enhance-Medical-Study.pdf

Lin, D. (2011, August 18). Parents Count on Stem Cells from Teeth. *NBC 4 Southern California*. Retrieved from http://www.nbclosangeles.com/news/health/Extracting-Stem-Cells-from-Your-Teeth-127799208.html

Medical News Today. (n.d.), Adult Stem Cells. Retrieved from http://www.medicalnewstoday.com/info/stem_cell/

Miller, J. (2010, July 27). When Milliseconds Mean Everything. *Wall Street Journal*. Retrieved from http://online.wsj.com/article/SB10001424052748703700904575391520412818094.html

Merriam-Webster (Definition of Aging), Retrieved from www.merriam-webster.com/dictionary/aging

Neporent, L. (2011, May 9). Stem Cells: Alternative to Knee
Replacement?. *ABC News*. Retrieved from
http://abcnews.go.com/Health/GMAHealth/stem-cell-
treatment-ease-osteoarthritis-pain-offer-
alternative/story?id=13550160

NewImageChannel. (2011, October 7). Oprah Regrown Finger
Video [Video file]. Retrieved from Youtube website:
http://www.youtube.com/watch?v=u3nl__psfBA

Nocera, M.D., R. (2011). *Cells That Heal Us From Cradle To
Grave*. Scottsdale, Arizona: Scottsdale Multimedia, Inc.

Nocera, M.D., R. (2011, March 28). Cells That Heal Us - Part
3 - Medistem: MEDSPK [Video file]. Retrieved from Youtube
website:
http://www.youtube.com/watch?v=vnvlfFVCOyE

Orlic, D., Kajstura, J., Chimenti, S., Jakoniuk I., Anderson
S.M., /Li, B,...Anversa, P. (2001, April 5). Bone Marrow
Cells Regenerate Infarcted Myocardium. *PubMed.gov*.
Abstract taken from *Nature* Retrieved from
http://www.ncbi.nlm.nih.gov/pubmed/11287958

Paddock, Ph.D., C. (2012, January 12). Type 1 Diabetes
Reversed With Stem Cells From Cord Blood. *Medical News
Today*. Retrieved from
http://www.medicalnewstoday.com/articles/240160.p
hp

Prentice, Ph.D., D. (2011, May 17). Adult Stem Cells are
Treating Thousands of Patients Now. *LifeNews.com*. Retrieved
from http://www.lifenews.com/2011/05/17/adult-
stem-cells-are-treating-thousands-of-patients-now/

Rath, M.D., M. (2001). *the Heart*. Santa Clara, California: MR Publishing, p. 44

Romereports. (2011, November 14). Pope gives support to adult stem cells and asks for ethics in scientific research. [Video file]. Retrieved from www.youtube.com website: http://www.youtube.com/watch?v=slKg9DZggu8

Reynolds, G. (2010, July 7). Phys. Ed: Your Brain on Exercise. *The New York Times*. Retrieved from http://well.blogs.nytimes.com/2010/07/07/your-brain-on-exercise/?src=me&ref=general

Schultheis, E. (2011, September 5). Rick Perry fires at Mitt Romney at S.C. town hall. *Politico*. Retrieved from http://www.politico.com/news/stories/0911/62649.html ScienceDaily: (2011, August 11).

Lasers Stimulate Stem Cells and Reduce Heart Scarring After Heart Attack, Study Says. *ScienceDaily*. Retrieved from http://www.sciencedaily.com/releases/2011/08/11081 1083820.htm

Senior Journal: (2010, December 1). Regular Exercise Increases Muscle Stem Cells to Renew Aging Muscles, Study Says. *Senior Journal*. Retrieved from http://baby seniorjournal.com/NEWS/Aging/2010/20101201-RegularExercise.htm

Soma@thehindu.co.in. (2012, April 8). Stem Cells market all set to grow: Study. *The Hindu Business Line*. Retrieved from http://www.thehindubusinessline.com/industry-and-economy/agri-biz/article3294059.ece?homepage=true&ref=wl_home

Steenblock, M.S., D.O., D., & Payne, Ph.D., A. (2006). *Umbilical Cord Stem Cell Therapy - The Gift of Newborns* . Laguna Beach, CA: Basic Health Publications Inc.

Taylor, R. (2011, October 25). Vatican Spends $1Million Promoting Adult Stem Cell Research. *LifeNews.com*. Retrieved from http://www.lifenews.com/2011 /10/25/vatican-spends-1-million-promoting-adult-stem-cell-research/?pr=1

Weisbart, P., & Weisbart, L. (2011). *Stillpoint Laser - Unwind and Dissolve Into Your Quantumfield*

Who discovered Penicillin?. (2012). In *info.com*. Retrieved from http://topics.info.com/Who-discovered-penicillin_214

Wikipedia. (220 types of cells), Retrieved from http://www.fact-index.com/b/bi/biological_cell.html

Winslow, R. (2010, March 9). To Double the Odds of Seeing 85: Get a Move On. *Wall Street Journal*. Retrieved from http://online.wsj.com/article/SB1000142405274870395 4904575109673558885594.html

Woodbury/Schwarz/Prockop/Black, D. (2000, August 15). Adult Rat and Human Bone Marrow Stromal Cells Differentiate into Neurons. *PubMed*.gov. Abstract taken from *Journal Neuroscience Research* Retrieved from http://www.ncbi.nlm.nih.gov/pubmed/10931522

XSilverX. (2011, February 3). The Skin Gun [Video file]. Retrieved from Youtube website: http://www.youtube.com/watch?v=7Y5H9Sasq5U

**REV UP YOUR ADULT STEM CELL POWER –
YOU NEED IT NOW!**

Young, R. (2012). U.S. Government as Purchaser of Stem Cell Therapies. *New York Stem Cell Summit 2012, 2012*, p. 7. Retrieved from http://www.stemcellsummit.com/StemCell_Fact_Sheet2012.pdf

Young, R. (2012). Stem Cell Use in the United States. *New York Stem Cell Summit*, p. 2. Retrieved from http://clients.criticalimpact.com/user/24825/files/StemCell_Fact_Sheet2012.pd

REV UP YOUR ADULT STEM CELL POWER –
YOU NEED IT NOW!

Notes:

REV UP YOUR ADULT STEM CELL POWER – YOU NEED IT NOW!

Notes:

REV UP YOUR ADULT STEM CELL POWER – YOU NEED IT NOW!

Notes:

Made in the USA
San Bernardino, CA
18 November 2015